NEUROSCIENCE RESEARCH PROGRESS

JOINT IMAGING APPLICATIONS IN GENERAL NEURODEGENERATIVE DISEASE

PARKINSON'S, FRONTOTEMPORAL, VASCULAR DEMENTIA AND AUTISM

NEUROSCIENCE RESEARCH PROGRESS

Additional books and e-books in this series can be found on Nova's website under the Series tab.

NEUROSCIENCE RESEARCH PROGRESS

JOINT IMAGING APPLICATIONS IN GENERAL NEURODEGENERATIVE DISEASE

PARKINSON'S, FRONTOTEMPORAL, VASCULAR DEMENTIA AND AUTISM

YONGXIA ZHOU, PHD

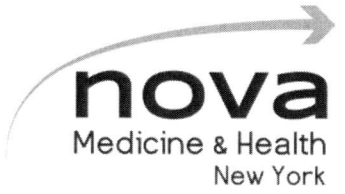

Copyright © 2021 by Nova Science Publishers, Inc.

All rights reserved. No part of this book may be reproduced, stored in a retrieval system or transmitted in any form or by any means: electronic, electrostatic, magnetic, tape, mechanical photocopying, recording or otherwise without the written permission of the Publisher.

We have partnered with Copyright Clearance Center to make it easy for you to obtain permissions to reuse content from this publication. Simply navigate to this publication's page on Nova's website and locate the "Get Permission" button below the title description. This button is linked directly to the title's permission page on copyright.com. Alternatively, you can visit copyright.com and search by title, ISBN, or ISSN.

For further questions about using the service on copyright.com, please contact:
Copyright Clearance Center
Phone: +1-(978) 750-8400   Fax: +1-(978) 750-4470   E-mail: info@copyright.com.

NOTICE TO THE READER

The Publisher has taken reasonable care in the preparation of this book, but makes no expressed or implied warranty of any kind and assumes no responsibility for any errors or omissions. No liability is assumed for incidental or consequential damages in connection with or arising out of information contained in this book. The Publisher shall not be liable for any special, consequential, or exemplary damages resulting, in whole or in part, from the readers' use of, or reliance upon, this material. Any parts of this book based on government reports are so indicated and copyright is claimed for those parts to the extent applicable to compilations of such works.

Independent verification should be sought for any data, advice or recommendations contained in this book. In addition, no responsibility is assumed by the Publisher for any injury and/or damage to persons or property arising from any methods, products, instructions, ideas or otherwise contained in this publication.

This publication is designed to provide accurate and authoritative information with regard to the subject matter covered herein. It is sold with the clear understanding that the Publisher is not engaged in rendering legal or any other professional services. If legal or any other expert assistance is required, the services of a competent person should be sought. FROM A DECLARATION OF PARTICIPANTS JOINTLY ADOPTED BY A COMMITTEE OF THE AMERICAN BAR ASSOCIATION AND A COMMITTEE OF PUBLISHERS.

Additional color graphics may be available in the e-book version of this book.

Library of Congress Cataloging-in-Publication Data

ISBN: 978-1-53619-435-7

Published by Nova Science Publishers, Inc. † New York

CONTENTS

Preface

Chapter 1 Functional Network and Coordination Deficits in Parkinson's Disease

Chapter 2 Molecular Imaging in Parkinson's Disease and PET/MRI Applications

Chapter 3 Fronto-Temporal Dementia: Imaging Biomarkers

Chapter 4 Vascular Dementia: Brain Structure and Function Evidence

Chapter 5 Multiparametric MRI Characterization in Autism Spectrum Disorder

About the Author

Index

PREFACE

Parkinson's disease (PD) is the second most prevalent neurodegenerative disorder with overall 0.2% prevalence rate; affecting 0.5-1% of individuals aged 65-69 years old and 1-3% for 80+ elderly people. The common signs include tremor, slowness of movement and rigidity; with occasionally neuropsychiatric problems such as depression, anxiety and apathy. In brain, the substantia nigra (SN) is the most early affected region causing decreased dopamine transmitter, with the possible basal ganglia-thalamo-cortical motor and other cognitive circuits involved. A few typical brain networks based on resting-state (RS)-fMRI had been investigated and were disrupted in PD patients including the sensorimotor network, the corticostriatal loop, thalamocortical and putamen-mesolimbic pathways; as well as the executive dysfunction of the frontoparietal network (FPN). Frontotemporal dementia (FTD) is another type of neurodegenerative disorder that has the frontal and temporal lobar abnormalities including atrophy and hypometabolism. The clinical impairments involve multiple domains such as executive function, memory, and emotion; with behavior variant (bv) as one primary type and two variants of primary progressive aphasia (PPA). Characteristic resting state network (RSN) abnormalities in bvFTD involved not only the salience network (mainly anterior cingulum, both ventral and dorsal portions), but also the default mode network (DMN) and FPN such as dorsolateral prefrontal cortex and precuneus that were associated with attention and working memory modulation.

Moreover, cerebral small vessel disease (SVD) is a leading cause of stroke that is a major source of morbidity and mortality in aging population. And stroke is reported to be a major cause of death (ranked 3rd) and long-term disability across the globe, with about half proportion of stroke survivors experiencing long-term dependency. Cerebral vasculature alterations including those affecting the subcortical white matter (WM) microcirculation might contribute to the cognitive impairment, commonly observed in Alzheimer's disease and stroke. It is expected that diffuse WM injury reflecting loss of myelin and axonal degeneration is one of the imaging hallmarks of vascular dementia (VaD), and atrophy of the medial temporal lobe including hippocampus with sclerosis is another feature of VaD. And finally, autism spectrum disorders (ASD) are a group of polygenetic developmental brain disorders with behavioral and cognitive impairment. Affected individuals exhibit stereotypical repetitive movements, restricted interests, lack of impulse control, speech deficits, impaired intelligence and social skills compared to typically developing (TD) children. Several studies revealed both structural and functional connectivity deficits in ASD including increased diffusivity and/or reduced fractional anisotropy in the long occipitofrontal fasciculus and interhemispheric corpus callosal (e.g., minor and major forceps) commissure, asymmetric and under-connected arcuate fasciculus language pathways, as well as reduced cerebellar-cortical interconnectivity. Functional connectivity of MRI (fcMRI) further identified abnormal disinhibition of some subcortical circuits, over- or under-connectivity in the superior temporal gyrus and amygdala.

Multiple advanced neuroimaging applications in various neurodegenerative diseases including PD, FTD, VaD and ASD are covered in this book. Relatively novel techniques such as integrated PET/MRI and combined independent component analysis and dual regression (ICA-DR) methods were developed to capture multi-level molecular/functional and structural/microstructural as well as high-order intra- and inter-network coordination abnormalities. For instance, consistent with the significantly lower values of diffusion tensor imaging (DTI) fractional anisotropy (FA) and fMRI voxel-mirrored homotopic correlation (VMHC) in the substantia nigra (swallow tail sign signature of PD), abrupt dopamine transporter (DAT) and striatal binding ratio (SBR) reductions in the caudate and putamen quantified with PET tracers were found in PD. VMHC deficits could possibly reflect demyelination (i.e., WM injury), discoordination (inter-network modulation), distance-based interhemispheric conductivity change (such as slowness of speed or response), and micro-structure related functional dysconnectivity at high sensitivity. Furthermore, the morphological atrophy, functional connectivity and conductivity deficits in PD revealed with MRI voxel based morphometry (VBM), VMHC and ICA-DR regions were co-localized with the decreased cortical vesicular monoamine transporter (VMAT2) densities in the bilateral mesial temporal cortex, caudate, orbitofrontal cortex, left frontal and occipital cortices identified by PET VMAT2 tracer for dopamine storage and pathway labeling. Similarly in FTD patients compared to normal controls (NC), the advanced MRI and fMRI methods such as VMHC and ICA-DR as well as PET molecular imaging data for amyloid accumulation and FDG glucose uptake identified typical brain atrophy, structural dis-connectivity, glucose hypometabolism, higher neuropathological burden, lower interhemispheric correlation together with functional dysconnectivity patterns in the orbitofrontal and anterior temporal cortices, with the cerebellum and dorsolateral prefrontal areas as compensation largely. In line with previous work, our MRI/PET results were consistent at multiple levels from molecular, metabolic, functional, structural, microstructural to brain circuits, and added multiparametric and comprehensive imaging evidence to the general clinical data cohort.

Functional and structural abnormalities had been further presented in the VaD dependent participants and the autistic children. For instance, both lower FA and VMHC, brain atrophy and functional connectivity deficits, demyelination, axonal degeneration and white matter integrity damage were present in the dependent compared to independent participants in VaD data cohort. Also increased neuronal activity with higher global mean values of fractional amplitude of low frequency fluctuation (fALFF) in the slow-wave sub-band S4 (0.027-0.073Hz) and conventional low frequency band (0.01-0.08Hz) were confirmed with less efficiency of systematic integration (i.e., lower global but higher local efficiency) based on small-worldness analysis in VaD dependent group. Furthermore, in ASD compared to controls, regional gray matter volume and cortical thickness in all four brain lobes increased, whereas white matter volume was decreased. In addition, lower functional connectivity in the temporal, visual and superior frontal regions but higher inferior and dorsolateral prefrontal cortical fcMRI were exhibited in ASD. The differentiation in each type of disease could also be revealed with the same imaging method based on either unique region/pattern and/or distinct brain circuit inter-connection, using VMHC, ICA-DR, DTI, VBM, fALFF and graph theory based small-worldness analysis. For instance, higher local efficiency in PD vs. NC, lower local efficiency but higher global efficiency in FTD vs. NC with closing eyes situation, both lower local and global efficiencies in FTD patients comparing opening to closing eyes relaxing conditions, higher local but lower global efficiencies in VaD-dependent patients vs. NC, and finally lower global efficiency in ASD vs. TD children were identified, indicating distinguishable disease-specific neuronal resource utilization and compensation strategy for each type of brain disorder.

Taken together, we had investigated neurodegenerative disease abnormalities in a more general and clinical perspective with multiparametric and multimodal imaging techniques. Our objective and confirmative results indicated great potential in utilizing these quantifications for accurate disease diagnosis and effective treatment. Unique imaging signature for each type and disease mechanism connection such as conductivity, inter-network correlation, systematic integration and efficiency analysis are the highlights of this book. The purpose of this book is thus to generalize and integrate conventional and advanced imaging methodologies for several common neurodegenerative diseases. With the thorough analysis and solid MRI/PET imaging results, this book would hope to capture the interests of readers in the broad fields of brain science and disease diagnosis. The author would like to specially thank the Alzheimer's disease neuroimaging initiative (ADNI) center at USC and several featured centers such as PPMI, NIFD, ABVIB and FCP, for providing the rich MRI/PET imaging data used in this book.

Specifically, Chapter 1 investigated MRI-based imaging abnormalities in several patient cohorts including PD and prodromal patients. Several advanced imaging techniques were introduced and applied, including VBM for brain atrophy, DTI for structural connectivity, RS-fMRI based VMHC for interhemispheric coordination and ICA-DR algorithm for multiple template matching and inter-network connectivity quantifications. For instance, reduced functional connectivity of multiple brain circuits in PD and prodromal patients compared to NC were identified with ICA-DR algorithm, including basal ganglia and temporal/orbitofrontal circuits, DMN and thalamic network, FPN, superior/medial frontal, temporal cortex and auditory networks. Network rerouting including hyper-connectivity in the motor, supplementary motor area, dorsolateral prefrontal and visual cortices were also present in the PD patients for functional compensation. The VMHC and ICA-DR metrics had been validated to be unique imaging biomarkers for PD patients with precise identification of disease abnormalities (such as the swallowing tail sign in substantia nigra together with typical intra- and inter- functional network alterations) and high correlations with other quantitative metrics as well as acceptable accuracy for classifying patients. As cross-validation and integration, PET molecular imaging data for dopamine transporter, binding potential and storage/pathway were analyzed in Chapter 2. The PET imaging results were in agreement with MRI results, demonstrated dramatically lower DAT and SBR levels in caudate/putamen (~50% reduction in PD) as well as lower cortical VMAT2 levels. More PET/MRI applications in brain science and neurological diseases were reviewed with another representative example, confirming the multiparametric quantification utilizing the integrated PET/MRI imaging for neurological and biological factor investigation.

Chapter 3 applied the similar MRI/PET methods for the FTD patients, as another neurodegenerative disease application example. Both the VMHC and ICA-DR results identified interhemispheric dis-coordination and multi-circuit dysregulation, with the RS-fMRI data acquired at several situations including baseline-longitudinal comparison in FTD patients, opening vs. closing eyes relaxing conditions for bvFTD together with the conventional bvFTD and NC comparison. These imaging abnormalities in the frontal and temporal regions together with insular and frontoparietal networks were more severe for opening compared to closing eyes relaxing conditions in patients, in contrast to the conventional comparisons between bvFTD and NC and least significant in the longitudinal comparison. Then Chapter 4 explored the disease mechanisms of VaD, especially the relatively severe case with higher risks in dependent living participants compared to independent living group, and revealed the brain abnormalities with multiparametric images. In addition to the previously mentioned advanced fMRI techniques, several DTI diffusivity metrics including axial and radial diffusivities reflecting axonal degeneration and demyelination, relatively new tract-based quantification and longitudinal analyses were performed. For instance, longitudinal changes of FA and diffusivity metrics together with alterations at each visit between two groups in certain brain tracts such as uncinate fasciculus and corticospinal tract for memory, movement and inhibition connectivity were identified, suggesting white matter integrity damage such as demyelination, axonal and Wallerian degeneration in the dependent group. Our results were consistent with previous reported findings in general VaD, and provided systematic, comprehensive and relatively new neuropathological clues to the disease severity. Finally, Chapter 5 employed volumetry, cortical thickness and functional connectivity based on MRI data to improve characterization and prediction of ASD. The results of increased gray matter volume, cortical thickness and reduced white matter volume as well as disrupted frontal and caudal functional connectivity in ASD compared to TD children were correlated with multiple clinical tests and phenotypic data, suggesting our imaging metrics could potentially serve as biomarkers in prognosis, diagnosis and disease progression monitoring.

Chapter 1 – Previous studies had reported brain regions such as substantia nigra (SN) and several circuits including motor and attentional network deficits in Parkinson's disease (PD) compared to controls. The purposes of this study are to: 1. use advanced fMRI data processing techniques including interhemispheric coordination with voxel-mirrored homotopic correlation (VMHC) as well as intrinsic network remapping with dual regression (DR) and independent component analysis (ICA) methods for multiple inter-network functional coordination computation to detect brain abnormalities in PD; 2. apply these techniques in another two patient cohorts with available data including prodromal (PM) patients, and PD from general cohort (GPD) with slightly more severity than PD; and 3. perform comprehensive analysis such as graph theory based small-worldness and classification evaluation as well as correlational quantification of various fMRI metrics. Both diffusion tensor imaging (DTI) and VMHC results revealed the swallow tail sign signature of SN in PD/GPD patients compared to normal controls (NC). Furthermore, the lower VMHC regions colocalized with the gray matter atrophy regions in patients, including inferior and middle temporal cortex, medial-orbito frontal cortex, dorsolateral prefrontal cortex, lingual, motor and supplementary motor cortices, as well as small regions in the posterior basal ganglia and cerebellum. Reduced functional connectivity of multiple brain circuits in PD/GPD/PM patients compared to NC were identified with ICA-DR algorithm including basal ganglia and temporal/orbitofrontal circuits, default mode network (DMN) and thalamic network, frontoparietal network, motor and supplementary motor circuits, superior/medial frontal, temporal cortex and auditory networks were identified. Network rerouting including hyper-connectivity in the motor, supplementary motor and dorsolateral prefrontal and visual cortices were also present in PD group, possibly for functional compensation. And global efficiency based on functional connectivity with small-worldness analysis was lower in PD patients with slightly higher local efficiency, resulting in higher small-worldness factor in patients compared to controls. Furthermore, global VMHC correlated with fractional amplitude of low frequency fluctuation (fALFF) and functional connectivity in the DMN and thalamus/putamen. Quantitative VMHC and ICA_DR had been validated to be unique imaging biomarkers for patients with precise identification of disease abnormalities and high correlations with other quantitative metrics as well as acceptable accuracy for classifying patients.

Chapter 2 – In addition to the previous MRI results of PD/GPD/PM in chapter 1, the purpose of Section I in this chapter is to reveal the PET molecular imaging abnormalities in these patients, including the dopamine transporter (DAT) and striatal binding ratio (SBR) data, as well as the vesicular monoamine transporter type 2 (VMAT2) with region-of-interest (ROI) based quantifications. Expected lower SBR and DAT levels in PD compared to NC were found in the striatal caudate and putamen regions. Generally less VMAT2 densities in PD/GPD compared to NC were found in the bilateral mesial temporal cortex, caudate, orbitofrontal cortex, left frontal and occipital cortices, however with a lower level in PM compared to other groups were observed additionally. The PET molecular imaging results, showing reduced dopamine transporter and binding potential levels in striatum and less cortical (spare of parietal lobe) and caudate dopamine storage and pathway deficits, were in line with the MRI imaging results including swallow tail sign (dopaminergic neuron reductions in nigrosome-1 territory) in substantia nigra with less microstructural connectivity or conductivity, gray matter atrophy and lower interhemispheric coordination/functional connectivity in the cortical inferior/middle temporal and medial-orbito frontal regions. Section II reviewed the multimodal PET/MRI applications in brain science and neurological diseases, and further elucidated PET/MRI combination for revealing the imaging differences affected with multiple physiological and neuropathological mechanisms. The representative example demonstrated the multiparametric quantification with the integrated PET/MRI imaging for the biological factor characterization.

Chapter 3 – Multiple brain networks were involved in frontotemporal dementia and mainly behavior variant type (bvFTD), that might be related to the brain atrophy and behavioral deficits in patients. The purposes of this work are to: 1. confirm the structural and functional connectivity differences in bvFTD patients using RS-fMRI and DTI data, and apply relatively new VMHC and ICA-DR methods for identifying interhemispheric dis-coordination and multi-circuit dysregulation in patients; 2. analyze the PET molecular imaging data for FDG-metabolism and amyloid neuropathological burden quantification and derive the statistical differences between patients and controls with PET imaging data; and 3. compare the differences of RS-fMRI data acquired at several conditions or between groups, including baseline-longitudinal analysis in FTD patients, opening vs. closing eyes conditions for bvFTD together with the conventional bvFTD vs. controls using brain stem as motion restriction. The advanced MRI and fMRI methods such as VMHC and ICA-DR as well as PET molecular imaging data identified the typical brain atrophy, hypometabolism, neuropathological burden as well as functional dysconnectivity patterns in the orbitofrontal and anterior temporal cortices, with the cerebellum and dorsolateral prefrontal areas as compensation largely. In line with previous work, our MRI/PET results were consistent at multiple levels from molecular, metabolic, functional, structural and microstructural to brain circuits, and added another perspective of comprehensive and multiparametric imaging evidence to the same data cohort.

Chapter 4 – Exploring the mechanisms of small vessel disease, especially the relatively severe case of vascular dementia (VaD, higher risks in dependent living participants compared to independent living), and reveal the effects of dependent living (in contrast to independent VaD participants) on the brain are one of the purposes of this study. Utilization of advanced imaging technique including relatively new tract-based white matter microstructural quantification and various diffusivity metrics as well as brain morphology and functional investigation at multiple levels, neural circuits and longitudinal visits is another goal. Our multiparametric imaging results demonstrated both structural and functional abnormalities in the dependent group compared to independent participants in the VaD data cohort, including lower FA, lower VMHC, brain atrophy and functional connectivity deficits in these patients. Increased global mean neuronal activity with higher fALFF in the slow-wave sub-band S4 and conventional low frequency band (0.01-0.08Hz) together with less efficiency of systematic integration (i.e., lower global but higher local efficiency) based on small-worldness analysis were also exhibited in dependent group compared to independent group. Furthermore, longitudinal changes of FA and diffusivity metrics together with alterations at each visit between two groups in certain brain tracts including cingulum, corticospinal tract and uncinate fasciculus for memory, movement and inhibition connectivity were present, suggesting white matter integrity damage such as demyelination, axonal and Wallerian degeneration in the dependent group. In addition to the agreement of each imaging finding, our systematic and relatively new results could provide neuropathological and neurophysiological clues to the disease severity in general VaD.

Chapter 5 – This study employed volumetry, cortical thickness and functional connectivity based on MRI data to improve characterization and prediction in autism spectrum disorders (ASD). Data from 127 children with ASD (13.5 ± 6.0 years) and 153 age- and gender-matched typically developing children (TD, 14.5 ± 5.7 years) were selected from the multi-center Functional Connectome Project. Regional gray matter volume and cortical thickness increased, whereas white matter volume decreased in ASD compared to TD children. Several disrupted functional connectivity of MRI (fcMRI) networks were also identified in ASD, including lower temporal, visual and superior frontal connectivity but higher inferior and dorsolateral prefrontal cortical fcMRI. Furthermore, volumetry and fcMRI were correlated with multiple clinical tests and phenotypic data, suggesting our imaging metrics could potentially serve as biomarkers in prognosis, diagnosis and disease progression monitoring.

Chapter 1

FUNCTIONAL NETWORK AND COORDINATION DEFICITS IN PARKINSON'S DISEASE

ABSTRACT

Previous studies had reported deficits in several brain regions such as substantia nigra (SN) and cortical circuits including motor and attentional network in Parkinson's disease (PD) compared to controls. The purposes of this study are to: 1. use advanced fMRI data processing techniques including interhemispheric coordination with voxel-mirrored homotopic correlation (VMHC) as well as intrinsic network remapping with dual regression (DR) and independent component analysis (ICA) methods for multiple intra- and inter-network functional coordination computation to detect brain abnormalities in PD; 2. apply these techniques in another two patient cohorts with available data including prodromal (PM) patients, and PD from general (GPD) cohort with slightly more severity than PD; and 3. perform comprehensive analysis such as graph theory based small-worldness and classification evaluation as well as correlational quantification of various fMRI metrics.

Both diffusion tensor imaging (DTI) and VMHC results revealed the swallow tail sign signature of SN in PD/GPD patients compared to normal controls (NC). Furthermore, the lower VMHC regions co-localized with the gray matter atrophy regions in patients, including inferior and middle temporal cortex, medial-orbito frontal cortex, dorsolateral prefrontal cortex, lingual, motor and supplementary motor cortices, as well as small regions in the posterior basal ganglia, right insular and cerebellum. Reduced functional connectivity of multiple brain circuits in PD/GPD/PM patients compared to NC were identified with ICA-DR algorithm including basal ganglia and temporal/orbitofrontal circuits, default mode network (DMN) and thalamic network, frontoparietal network, motor and supplementary motor circuits, superior/medial frontal, temporal cortex and auditory networks were identified. Network rerouting including hyper-connectivity in the motor, supplementary motor and dorsolateral prefrontal and visual cortices were also present in PD group, possibly for functional compensation. And global efficiency based on functional connectivity with small-worldness analysis was lower in PD patients with slightly higher local efficiency, resulting in higher small-worldness factor in patients compared to controls. Furthermore, global VMHC correlated with fractional amplitude of low frequency fluctuation (fALFF) and functional connectivity in the DMN and thalamus/putamen. Quantitative VMHC and ICA_DR had been validated to be unique imaging biomarkers for PD with precise identification of disease abnormalities and high correlations with other quantitative metrics as well as acceptable accuracy for classifying patients.

Keywords: dual regression, independent component analysis, voxel-mirrored homotopic correlation, Parkinson's disease, prodromal stage, fractional amplitude of low frequency fluctuation, brain circuit, substantia nigra, basal ganglia, swallow tail sign, striatum, motor cortex, supplementary motor area, nigrosome-1, diffusion tensor imaging, tremor, default mode network, thalamus, frontoparietal network, dorsolateral attentional network, dorsolateral prefrontal cortex, insula, movement disorder, small-worldness, efficiency, gray matter atrophy, voxel-based morphometry

1. INTRODUCTION

Morphometry analysis of Parkinson's disease (PD) had identified brain atrophy in both subcortical and cortical regions including the basal ganglia, basal forebrain, midbrain and medial temporal lobe [1]. Also these abnormalities were predictive of the longitudinal clinical symptom progression [2]. Especially, the loss of nigrosome-1 (N1) (dopaminergic neurons in the N1 territory) in the substantia nigra (SN) is one of the imaging hallmarks of PD. The increase of paramagnetic iron in the SN could be visualized with magnetic resonance imaging (MRI) $T2^*$-weighted iron-sensitive sequences including conventional functional MRI (fMRI) and quantitative susceptibility mapping (QSM) [3]. Functional neuroimaging studies had reported the nigrostriatal degeneration that could help understand the pathophysiology of the disease [4]. For instance, basal ganglia network connectivity dysfunction could reflect dopamine transportation differences in both sleep behavior disorder and PD that might help disease early prevention [5]. Furthermore, the hyper-connectivity (or hyper-synchronization) between basal ganglia and cortical motor network was often observed in PD, suggesting altered basal-cortical motor control and possible compensatory role in patients [6]. Lower neuronal activity in the striatum, middle frontal and occipital cortices as well as supplementary motor area (SMA) together with higher activity in the cerebellum, thalamus, superior parietal lobule (part of the motor network) and precuneus had been reported and seemed to validate the compensatory mechanism [7].

Controversial results had been reported for conventional seed-based method regarding the resting-state functional connectivity (RSFC) networks. For instance, it was reported that the SN had decreased connectivity in the striatum, globus pallidus, subthalamic nucleus, thalamus, SMA, dorsolateral prefrontal cortex (DLPFC), insula, default mode network (DMN), temporal lobe, cerebellum and pons in patients compared to controls [8]. However it was later found that these PD-related functional connectivity changes turned out to be non-reproducible across datasets, and the discrepancy could be due to disease heterogeneity and individual variability [9]. A more advanced intrinsic data-based independent component analysis (ICA) had identified reliably both PD-related and cognition-related resting-state (RS)-fMRI patterns that were similar to the metabolic PET images [10]. A few typical brain networks based on RS-fMRI had been investigated and were disrupted in PD patients including the sensorimotor network, the corticostriatal loop, thalamocortical and putamen-mesolimbic pathways; as well as the executive dysfunction of the frontoparietal network (FPN) [11, 12]. Dysconnectivity of these networks such as hypoactivity in the frontal and parietal hubs was associated with the decline of cognitive performances including hallucinations and visual misperceptions, as well as insular atrophy that was related to the attentional network deficits [13].

Inter- and intra- network variability and correlation differences in PD compared to controls had been investigated and results were further correlated to cognitive dysfunction. For instance, time-varying of the RSFC (individual abnormalities) of DMN, attention and executive function networks were related to the worse clinical assessments [14]. As expected, PD patients also presented larger intra-network variation including the salience, visual and subcortical networks [15]. The inter-network connectivity was reduced in patients between the dorsal attentional network (DAN) including DLPFC and salience networks, and was associated with the misperception scores in PD [16]. In addition, the increased inter-correlation between insular network and DMN in PD was correlated with the lower attentional accuracy [17]. And machine learning algorithm using the whole-brain connectivity RS-fMRI data presented good accuracy of ~80% for classifying PD patients from controls [18]. Finally, the integration of brain network organization reported decreased global efficiency with increased local efficiency in PD compared to controls based on RS-fMRI functional connectivity [19].

Previous studies had reported brain regions such as SN and several circuits including motor and attentional network deficits in PD compared to controls. The purposes of this study are to: 1. using advanced MRI and fMRI data processing technique including interhemispheric coordination and intrinsic network remapping for intra- and inter-network correlation examination with relatively novel methods such as dual regression and independent component analysis methods to detect brain functional and structural abnormalities in PD; 2. apply these techniques in two other patient cohorts with available data including prodromal patients and PD from general cohort with slightly more severity than PD; and 3. perform further comprehensive analyses such as graph theory based small-worldness and classification evaluation as well as statistical correlational quantification for various fMRI metrics.

2. METHODS

2.1. Participants and Data Acquisitions

MRI/PET Imaging data used in the preparation of this article were obtained from the ADNI database (http://ida.loni.usc.edu). The primary goal of ADNI has been to test whether serial MRI, positron emission tomography (PET), other biological markers, and clinical and neuropsychological assessment can be combined to measure the progression of mild cognitive impairment (MCI) and early Alzheimer's disease (AD). ADNI is the result of efforts of many co-investigators from a broad range of academic institutions and private corporations, and subjects have been recruited from over 50 sites across the United States and Canada. For up-to-date information, see www.adni-info.org.

Specifically, all participants were recruited and managed in the Parkinson's Progression Markers Initiative (PPMI) program as one featured ADNI center that contains and manages the full set of imaging and clinical data. Available and most recent fMRI imaging data of four sub-groups were downloaded and processed. The unified Parkinson's disease rating scale (UPDRS) score was obtained from all participants for assessing motor and tremor related function. As listed in Table 1, resting-state (RS)-fMRI data from 19 Parkinson's disease (PD) patients (age: 66.4 ± SD 2.3 years, UPDRS score = 31.3 ± 2.2, 6 women), 7 PD from general cohort (GPD) (age: 63.9 ± SD 1.7 years, UPDRS score = 33.3 ± 3.8, 2 women), 4 prodromal (PM) patients (age: 66.3 ± SD 1.4 years, UPDRS score = 15.5 ± 9.5, 1 women) and 8 age-matched normal controls (NC) from general cohort unaffected individuals (age: 64.8 ± SD 4.0 years, UPDRS score = 2.1 ± 1.0, 5 women) were processed further. As expected, the UPDRS was significantly higher in PD and GPD groups compared to NC (both $P \leq 0.0001$). There were no other significant UPDRS differences between pairs of sub-groups, with trend of higher score in PM group compared to NC and lower score in PM compared to PD/GPD group, possibly due to the relatively small number of participants and large variation in PM group.

Table 1. Demographic information of subjects in four groups of the PD data cohort

Group	Age (Years)	Women n/%	Total N	UPDRS	P-value (UPDRS) of two sub-group comparisons
1-NC	64.8 ± 4.0	5/63%	8	2.1 ± 1.0	0.2545 (NC,PM)
2-PM	66.3 ± 1.4	1/25%	4	15.5 ± 9.5	**< 0.0001 (NC,PD)**
3-PD	66.4 ± 2.3	6/32%	19	31.3 ± 2.2	**0.0001 (NC,GPD)**
4-GPD	63.9 ± 1.7	2/29%	7	33.3 ± 3.8	0.1577 (PM,GPD)

* PD = Parkinson's disease, GPD = PD from general cohort, PM = prodromal stage, NC = normal controls from unaffected general cohort. Last column indicated P-value comparing UPDRS scores between two sub-groups.

The UPDRS motor scores were significantly higher in PD and GPD patients compared to controls (both $P \leq 0.0001$). There were no significant differences of UPDRS score in other sub-group comparisons, with a trend of lower UPDRS in prodromal (PM) patients than PD and GPD. For instance, $P = 0.26$ comparing PM group to NC and $P = 0.16$ comparing PM to GPD group. The other two comparisons of UPDRS score were: P(PM, PD) = 0.1957 and P(PD, GPD) = 0.6553.

2.2. Imaging Parameters and Data

All MRI experiments were performed using the 3T scanner with standardized imaging protocols. For the resting-state (RS)-fMRI data, a standard gradient-echo EPI sequence (TR/TE = 2400/25 msec, flip angle = 80°, number of volumes = 210, spatial resolution = 3.3 x 3.3 x 5.0 mm^3) was performed. The 3D MPRAGE (TR/TE/TI = 2300/900/2.9 ms, flip angle = 9°, matrix size = 256 x 256 x 176, resolution = 1 x 1x 1 mm^3) was also obtained for structural and morphological analysis such as gray matter atrophy, as well as the reference image and anatomical normalization of seed-based fMRI functional connectivity and coordination data.

Preprocessed diffusion tensor imaging (DTI) data in the substantia nigra region were downloaded from the ADNI website for validation. A total of 8 sub-regions including left and right sides of the three portions of substantia nigra (rostral, middle and caudal segments) and cerebral peduncle as the reference were evaluated between patients and controls with the DTI fractional anisotropy (FA) metric.

2.2.1. MRI Image and Processing

Using FMRIB Software Library (FSL, http://www.fmrib.ox.ac.uk/fsl) toolbox, voxel based morphometry (VBM) algorithm was performed to the structural MPRAGE data for brain atrophy quantification. The processing steps involved tissue segmentation of gray matter, white matter and cerebrospinal fluid (CSF), spatial normalization to the FSL 2mm template with nonlinear warping, spatial modulation and smoothing. And finally statistical analysis with non-parametric permutation was implemented to detect gray matter density differences between patients and controls or each pair of two sub-groups.

The RS-fMRI data were preprocessed with motion correction and outlier screening such as mean frame displacement (FD) < 0.6 mm to remove excessive motion. We used 3D high resolution T1-MPRAGE for image coregistration and normalization. To generate functional connectivity of MRI (fcMRI) map using seed-based analysis, Pearson's correlation between the preprocessed average time series of the pre-selected seed (region of interest or specific network pattern) and each voxel within the whole brain area was computed. The resultant values of Z-transformed (using Fisher's r-to-z transform) map were used for subsequent group-level post-hoc statistical analysis [22].

2.2.2. VMHC

Previous work had reported that the interhemispheric functional coordination and integration plays an important role in communicating, motor function, cognitive, learning, attention and information processing [23]. We had also elucidated neurobiological and functional/ microstructural connections of the clinical symptoms and neurocognitive measures of various neurodegenerative patients using voxel-mirrored homotopic correlation (VMHC) technique that parallels to the myelin map and reflects structural conductivity between two brain hemispheres [24]. Briefly, VMHC was computed as the interhemispheric synchrony or voxel-mirrored hemispheric correlation after preprocessing RS-fMRI, similar to the voxel-wise fcMRI computation steps. The resultant correlational values were z-transformed (by use of the Fisher r-to-z transform) and were used for subsequent group- level analysis. We used a 2-sample Student t test to compare VMHC between the patient group and the healthy control group or each sub-group of patients such as PD vs. GPD. Multiple comparison corrections at the cluster level were performed to the whole brain based on Gaussian random field theory by the FSL easythresh command (minimum $Z > 2.3$; cluster significance, $P < 0.05$, corrected). The global VMHC score for each participant was obtained by averaging of the individual VMHC z-image of each participant within the 25% gray matter mask from the FSL template for further statistical comparison and correlational quantification [25].

2.2.3. RSFC and fALFF

Conventional resting state functional connectivity (RSFC) maps were generated from a total of 26 seeds consisting of the combined default mode network (DMN) core seed, 12 extensively used typical functional networks including regions of different sub-areas of DMN (e.g., posterior cingulate cortex and intra-parietal sulcus), 3 thalamic (left, right, and whole thalamus) and 7 thalamic segmental seeds for different brain lobar projections together with 3 subcortical seeds (caudate and putamen from the MNI template, and hypothalamus from an in-house developed probability map) [26]. The typical networks from 12 seeds were derived from the script seed library (http://www.nitrc.org/ projects/fcon_1000), including the hippocampal formation and frontal eye field (FEF) seeds that generated the task-positive networks (i.e., these networks are more active at task-conditions, in contrast to resting state). All seeds were well-evaluated and validated in our previous work [22, 26]. The global mean z-values and difference image were obtained from the fcMRI maps generated from each of 26 seeds to derive the intra-network differences statistically, by averaging and comparing the mean fcMRI Z-maps over the whole brain with a threshold of GRF cluster-corrected P < 0.01 between two subject groups.

In addition to fcMRI, the factional amplitude of low frequency fluctuation (fALFF) was calculated from RS-fMRI to reflect the intensity of regional spontaneous brain activity or neuronal activation. The idea of the fALFF method was to scale the summary of amplitude at the low-frequency band (e.g., 0.01–0.08 Hz) to the summary of amplitude across the whole frequency of the time course of each voxel to remove white and physiological noise [27]. fALFF values of additional two low frequency sub-bands including slow-waves of S5 (0.01-0.027 Hz) and S4 (0.027-0.073 Hz) were also evaluated for possible intrinsic motor and neuronal activity integration related alterations. About 12 data points in the periodic power spectrum fell in the slow wave S5 band, and another 11 points in the slow wave S4 band; with a total of about 24 data points in the conventional low-frequency band spectrum for fractional amplitude computation.

2.2.4. Dual Regression

Some relatively new methods including independent component analysis (ICA) with dual regression (ICA-DR) algorithm and graph theory based small-worldness network analysis were performed as well for further functional and systematic investigation [22, 28-29]. Independent component analysis (ICA) is a more robust technique involving the blind source separation method that captures the essential components of multivariate resting-state functional MR imaging data and removes the noise components. We had previously validated our RSFC findings using three different strategies of ICA, template-based ICA method, hybrid ICA seed-based method and group ICA method, in patients with mild traumatic brain injury compared with healthy individuals with the advanced automatic detection algorithm for component selection [22].

Intrinsic network-based dual regression (DR) model was applied to the ICA identified 20 networks from the template of resting state networks after preprocessing the RS-fMRI data. These validated 20 ICA-networks consisted of the four brain lobes (1 frontal network, 1 temporal, 1 auditory and 3 visual networks) in addition to 1 corticostriatal and 1 cerebellar-basal ganglia networks, as well as 4 well-known brain hubs including DMN, FPN, motor-sensory network and thalamo-cortical connectivity with 3 sub-networks for each hub [28]. The detailed ordering and function for the DR components of these 10 categorical remapped templates for both intra- and inter- network connectivity computations are listed below:

1) DR1, DR2, DR3: visual networks consisting of several sub-networks of different regions such as lingual, calcarine, precuneus and cuneus
2) DR4, DR10, DR12: thalamo-cortical networks with visual, cerebellum, temporal, frontal sub-networks
3) DR5: corticostriatal network including caudate, medial orbitofrontal and anterior temporal regions
4) DR6, DR13, DR14: posterior, anterior portions and typical whole DMN
5) DR7: cerebellum and basal ganglia
6) DR8, DR11, DR20: left, right and whole fronto-parietal networks (FPN)
7) DR9, DR15, DR19: motor, sensory and supplementary motor networks
8) DR16: auditory cortex, insula and anterior cingulate (salience network)
9) DR17: frontal network including DAN and DLPFC
10) DR18: temporal network including inferior parietal lobe

The ICA-DR model could separate complex functional networks by dual template matching, including 1st-level multiple intra-network templates generated from initial ICA decomposition as seeds and 2nd-level regression analysis for inter-network template-pattern re-mapping computation. Namely, ICA-based DR could be used to investigate the dual-level intra- and inter-network connections with multiple initial ICA-identified template networks. Compared to conventional RSFC, similar to the hybrid ICA seed-based method, ICA-DR model enhanced the detection sensitivity of both intra-network connectivity and complicate inter-network coordination with more convergent and complementary spatial information as well as higher signal to noise ratio (SNR) [22, 26, 28].

2.2.5. Small-Worldness Property Characterization

To understand the whole-brain functional network integration and specialization, small-worldness analyses were performed on the preprocessed fcMRI data. A few key terminologies commonly used in graph theory and this work include (1) degree (D), which is equal to the number of connections (edges) attached to each node or region of interest (ROI); (2) clustering coefficient (C_p) which measures the number of connections of a node with its nearest nodes (neighbors), namely, the fraction of the number of a node's neighbors that are also neighbors of each other, reflecting how efficiently the network exchanges the information at the cluster level; (3) betweenness centrality (BC), which measures the number of shortest paths between pairs of other nodes that pass through the node, reflecting how efficiently the network exchanges the information at the global level; (4) Path length (L_p), which computes the length of the shortest path between a pair of nodes, is another measure of global efficiency. BC is high for nodes that are located on many short paths in the network and low for nodes that do not participate in many short paths and are therefore more peripheral; on the other hand, longer L_p indicates worse global efficiency; and (5) core number (K) which is defined as the largest k such that the node is still contained in the kth-core (the largest subgraph comprising nodes of degree at least k), reflecting the rigidity or stability of the network [29-31].

Using the fMRI data after pre-processing, the Pearson correlation between every pair of ROIs of a whole-brain parcellation was computed to derive the original correlation matrix for each subject after the time courses were extracted and averaged over each ROI. An atlas with a total of 112 ROIs covering the entire cerebrum including cortical and subcortical regions was used as whole-brain parcellation [23, 26]. A threshold r value of 0.2 to 0.95 was applied to this correlation matrix to investigate the small-worldness measures at different sparsity levels. The binarized correlation matrix was used for small-worldness analyses, including absolute clustering coefficients (C_p) and path lengths (L_p). A random network with the same number of degrees as the real network (i.e., the correlation matrix) was generated and used as a scaling factor to compute the relative local efficiency ($\gamma = C_p/C_{p\text{-random}} >> 1$) and global efficiency ($\lambda = L_p/L_{p\text{-random}} \approx 1$) at different sparsity levels. The global small-worldness factor ($\sigma = \gamma/\lambda$) was also derived.

2.2.6. Correlational Analysis and Classification

The statistical correlation between global mean VMHC and fALFF Z-values, as well as correlations between VMHC/fALFF and global RSFC network functional connectivity strength were further quantified.

Classifier performance was evaluated with accuracy (ACC), sensitivity (SEN), specificity (SPE) and positive predictive value (PRE) using the global VMHC Z-value imaging feature [32]. To compare results of multiple classifiers and choose the best one, the default support vector machine (SVM) classifier with quadratic fitting (QP), k-means nearest-neighbor (KNN) classifier, SVM classifiers with other kernel functions such as radial basis function (RBF) and polynomial function mapping were implemented. And the classifier with the best performance was used for the final result. Two criteria including average and maximum were used for selection in the iterations for either four groups including PD, NC, GPD and PM; or conventional classification including only two groups of PD and NC. The optimal performance of each classifier was obtained by extracting the maximum value out of 1000 iterations and the average performance was also achieved for all iterations. All results were evaluated with 5-fold cross-validation (CV).

3. RESULTS

Significantly higher FD, especially in the mean top quartile (P = 0.0015) and mean top decile (P = 0.0017) were detected in the PD patients compared to controls (Table 2). The mean and root mean square (RMS) error of FD were also higher in PD patients, with marginal significance in RMS metric (P = 0.0462) and a trend in the mean FD metric (P = 0.130). Similar FD differences were also found in GPD patients compared to NC, with a trend in PM group as well.

Significantly lower FA in the right substantia nigra (middle portion) was detected in PD patients compared to NC (P = 0.008), indicating swallow tail sign signature of Parkinson's disease (Table 3). Slightly higher FA in the right cerebral peduncle region was found however, possibly due to the relatively less radial space and therefore more axonal integrity in PD.

Table 2. RS-fMRI data motion quantification with frame displacement (FD) and difference between PD and NC

Comparison	Mean FD	RMS FD	Mean Top Quartile FD	Mean Top Decile FD
NC	0.8272 ± 0.1785	0.9465 ± 0.2107	1.4173 ± 0.3157	1.3547 ± 0.3188
PD	1.2249 ± 0.1781	1.4179 + 0.2164	2.1906 ± 0.3388	2.0338 ± 0.2939
P(NC, PD)	0.1303	0.0462	0.0015	0.0017

*RMS=root of mean square of difference.

Table 3. ROI-based DTI FA evaluation showing significant FA reduction in the right middle portion of basal ganglia (ROI4, P = 0.0075) comparing PD to NC group

ROI	NC	PD	P-value
ROI4	0.322 ± 0.008	0.297 ± 0.005	0.0075
REF2	0.600 ± 0.007	0.614 ± 0.003	0.0359

*ROI4 = right middle substantia nigra region (size = 30mm^3); REF2 = right cerebral peduncle as reference region.

VBM structural results demonstrated gray matter atrophy in PD patients compared to controls in the clusters in inferior and middle temporal cortex, medial-orbito frontal cortex, dorsolateral prefrontal cortex, right insula, motor and supplementary motor cortices. On the other hand, small regions in cerebellum, left insula, posterior putamen and basal ganglia also presented higher gray matter density in PD patients (Figure 1A, P<0.05). Lower interhemispheric coordination detected with VMHC maps in the basal ganglia including the swallow tail signs in the substantia nigra, red nucleus, hypothalamus, thalamus, ventral striatum, caudate, lingual gyrus, postcentral gyrus, frontal pole and temporal cortex were found in PD compared to NC (Figure 1B, P<0.001). A few regions in the middle and superior frontal cortices, middle cingulate, fusiform, motor cortex and supplementary motor area, superior parietal lobe and primary visual cortex also showed higher VMHC values, reflecting functional coordination or coherence abnormalities in PD patients compared to controls. Quantitative significant differences in large brain clusters with P < 0.01 are listed in Table 4.

Table 4. Significant VMHC differences comparing PD to NC groups with P < 0.01. Brain clusters on one side are listed due to the symmetrical interhemispheric computation

Brain Clusters	Cluster Size	P-value	MAX Z score	MAX X(vox)	MAX Y(vox)	MAX Z(vox)
A. Regions showing decreased VMHC in PD patients compared to NC (P < 0.01)						
Frontal Pole	5305	< 1.0E-34	10.7	30	94	28
Postcentral Gyrus	3224	8.9E-34	8.19	39	45	72
Hippocampus	914	1.6E-13	8.46	33	54	26
Occipital Pole	327	6.5E-06	8.54	33	13	29
Inferior Temporal Gyrus	250	0.00012	5.78	19	48	23
Caudate	201	0.00091	8.36	40	64	42
Lingual-fusiform Gyrus	193	0.00129	5.32	34	34	32
Lingual Gyrus	173	0.00310	7.39	40	33	35
Temporal Pole	154	0.00740	8.15	34	70	18
B. Regions showing increased VMHC in PD patients compared to NC (P < 0.01)						
Primary Visual Cortex	21553	< 1.0E-34	14.6	39	18	27
Medial Prefrontal Cortex	319	8.7E-06	9.52	37	93	36
Superior Parietal Lobe	149	0.00934	6.51	33	34	56

Comparison of VMHC images between GPD and NC (Figure 2, P<0.001) showed similar results as in Figure 1B (PD vs. NC). However, less degree of lower VMHC but more higher or positive regions in GPD compared to NC were identified as shown in Figure 2A and B (GPD vs.

NC and GPD vs. PD statistical comparisons respectively). The positive regions with higher functional coordination in GPD patients compared to NC and PD included clusters in superior parietal and occipital cortices such as lingual, orbitofrontal cortex, fusiform and inferior temporal cortex.

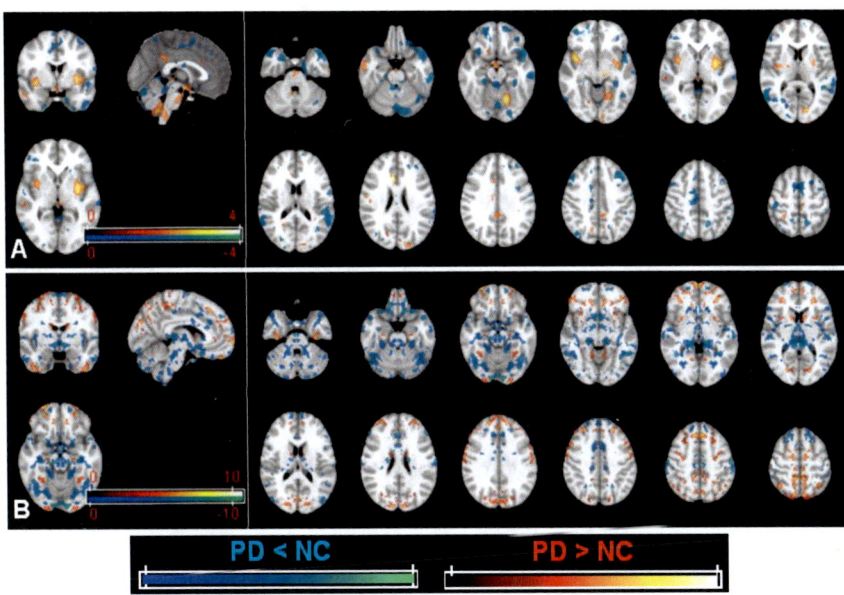

Figure 1. A: VBM results showing gray matter atrophy in patients; red: PD > NC; blue: PD < NC (P < 0.05); B: VMHC showing interhemispheric correlation differences; red: PD > NC, blue: PD < NC (P < 0.001). Gray matter atrophy in PD patients compared to controls in multiple clusters of inferior and middle temporal cortex, medial-orbito frontal cortex, dorsolateral prefrontal cortex, motor and supplementary motor cortices, as well as small regions in the posterior basal ganglia, right insula and cerebellum were identified (blue color in A). On the other hand, small regions in inferior cerebellum, left insula, calcarine, medial hypothalamus, posterior putamen and basal ganglia-red nucleus area also presented higher gray matter density in PD patients (red color in A). Lower interhemispheric coordination in the temporal cortex, basal ganglia including the swallow tail signs in the substantia nigra, red nucleus, hypothalamus, thalamus, ventral striatum, caudate, lingual gyrus, precentral gyrus, rectus, and temporal cortex regions were found in PD compared to NC (blue color in B). A few regions in the middle and superior frontal, middle cingulate, fusiform, motor and supplementary motor cortices, superior parietal and occipital cortices also showed higher functional coordination in PD patients compared to controls (red color in B).

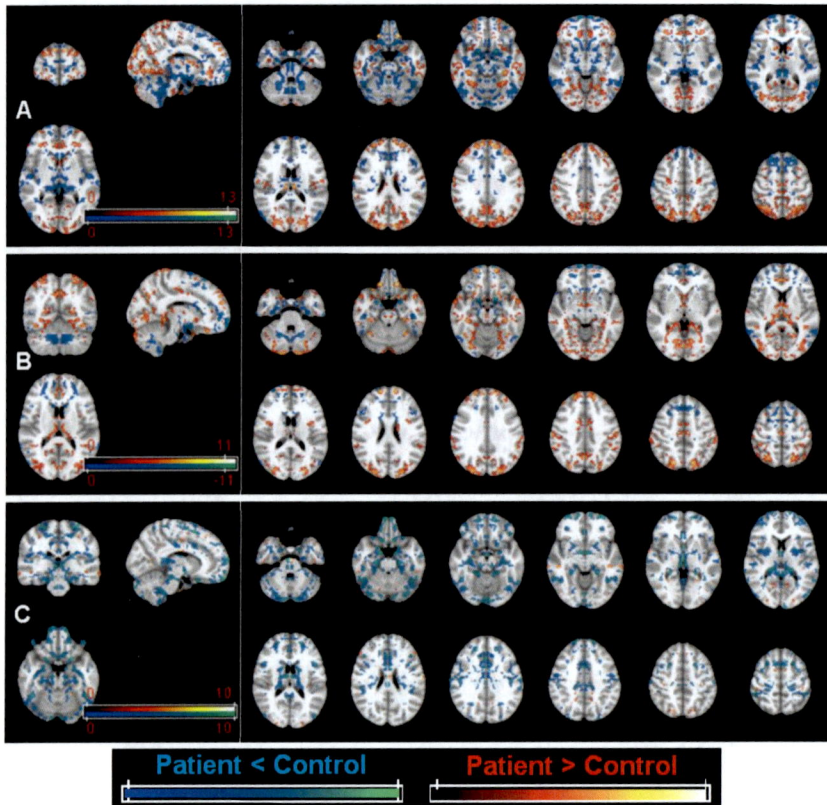

Figure 2. VMHC map comparisons between sub-groups including GPD and prodromal (PM) groups in addition to PD and NC with P<0.001. A: GPD vs. NC; blue: GPD<NC, red: GPD > NC. B: GPD vs. PD; blue: GPD < PD, red: GPD > PD. C: Prodromal (PM) vs. NC; blue: PM<NC, red: PM > NC. Similarly lower VMHC regions in GPD compared to NC (blue color in A) were found in the basal ganglia including substantia nigra and red nucleus, temporal cortex including hippocampus, middle frontal and supplementary motor cortex as in Figure 1B blue color. And mostly lower VMHC values were identified in the basal ganglia, ventro-medial hypothalamus, posterior putamen, distributed clusters in the temporal and orbitofrontal cortices such as hippocampus and amygdala, motor and supplementary regions, as well as middle and superior frontal cortices in PM compared to NC groups as in C.

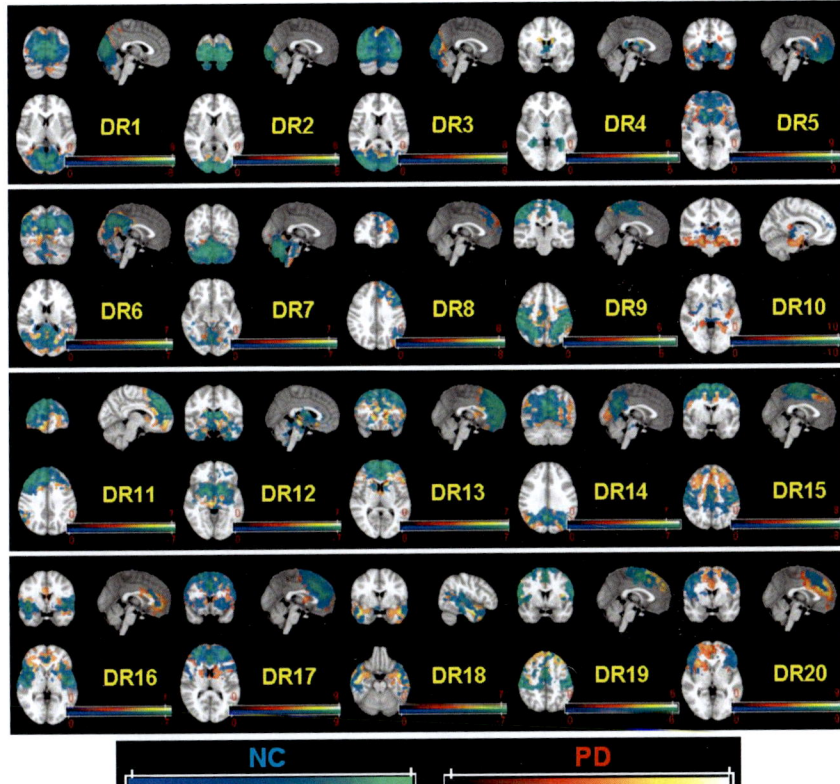

Figure 3. Dual regression patterns and comparisons between PD and NC. A total of 20 network-based regressors from ICA decomposition template were applied for intra- and inter-network remapping, and mean results of each group were demonstrated with P < 0.01. Blue-green for control group and overlapped with the red-orange color for PD group. The 10 categories of all 20 ICA-DR components were:
1) DR1, DR2, DR3: visual networks such as lingual, calcarine, precuneus and cuneus
2) DR4, DR10, DR12: thalamo-cortical networks with visual, temporal and frontal
3) DR5: corticostriatal network including caudate, medial orbito-frontal and anterior temporal regions
4) DR6, DR13, DR14: posterior, anterior portions and typical whole DMN
5) DR7: cerebellum and basal ganglia
6) DR8, DR11, DR20: left, right and whole fronto-parietal networks (FPN)
7) DR9, DR15, DR19: motor, sensory and supplementary motor networks
8) DR16: auditory cortex, insula and anterior cingulate (salience network)
9) DR17: frontal network including DAN and DLPFC
10) DR18: temporal network including inferior parietal lobe
In this PD data cohort, the most significant inter-network correlation differences among these networks included component DR10-thalamic network, DR15-motor and supplementary motor network, DR20-FPN including dorsolateral prefrontal cortex, DR18-temporal cortex and DR16-auditory network.

Similarly, lower VMHC regions in GPD comparison to NC were found in the basal ganglia including substantia nigra and red nucleus, temporal cortex including hippocampus, middle frontal and supplementary motor cortex. Regarding the prodromal (PM) group vs. NC comparison in Figure 2C, mostly lower VMHC values existed in patients with small regions in basal ganglia, ventro-medial hypothalamus and posterior putamen, together with distributed clusters in temporal and orbitofrontal cortices, motor and supplementary regions as well as middle and superior frontal cortices.

No significant differences of conventional seed-based functional connectivity maps with RSFC method comparing four groups were found ($P > 0.05$). A total of 20 ICA template-based networks were identified, and used as 2nd-level inter-network remapping in ICA-DR algorithm. The average maps of each ICA-DR network pattern of PD and NC groups were demonstrated with $P < 0.001$ in Figure 3. The most significant differences among these networks included components DR10-thalamic network, DR15-motor and supplementary motor network, DR20-FPN including DLPFC, DR18-temporal cortex and 16-auditory network such as insular, superior temporal and anterior cingulate cortices.

For detailed ICA-DR between-group statistical comparisons, lower network connectivity with multi-slice views in the DMN regions (DR4 blue color) and subcortical caudate and thalamus regions (DR7), basal ganglia and temporal/orbitofrontal regions in DR8, motor regions in DR5, as well as SMA and FPN including superior/medial frontal regions in DR10 were observed in PD patients compared to controls ($P < 0.01$) (Figure 4). On the other hand, higher functional connectivity (positive or over-connectivity) in the regions of inter-frontal and motor/supplementary cortices in DR8, thalamo-cortical and dorsal attentional networks (DR5, DR6), temporal and occipital regions in DR7, DR6 and DR4, basal ganglia related motor region in DR7, together with supplementary motor cortex and occipital regions in DR9 existed in patients compared to controls, possibly for functional compensation (Figure 4). Furthermore, lower connectivity in the basal ganglia, visual cortex, FPN, motor and supplementary motor areas as well as cerebellum were confirmed in PD patients in most of later DR components (11th-20th) compared to controls (Figure 5; P < 0.01).

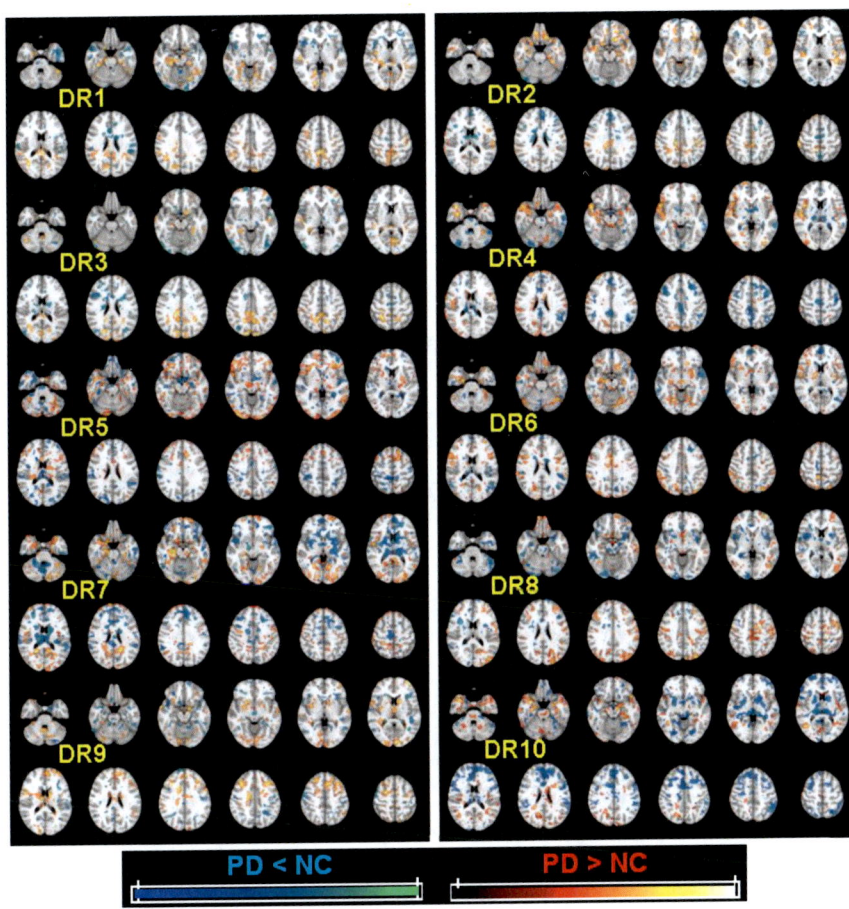

Figure 4. Statistical comparison map between PD and NC with P < 0.01 for the first 1-10 dual regression components (DR1-DR10). Red: PD > NC and Blue: PD < NC. Lower functional connectivity in the default mode network regions (DR4 blue color) and subcortical caudate and thalamus regions (DR7), regions in DR8, motor regions in DR5, as well as supplementary motor cortex and FPN in DR10 were observed in PD patients compared to controls (P < 0.01). On the other hand, higher connectivity (positive or over-connectivity) in the regions of motor and supplementary cortices in DR8 (red color), DAN, thalamocortical and dorsolateral prefrontal networks (DR5, DR6), temporal and occipital regions in DR7, DR6 and DR4, basal ganglia related motor region in DR7, together with supplementary motor cortex and occipital regions in DR9 were identified in patients compared to controls.

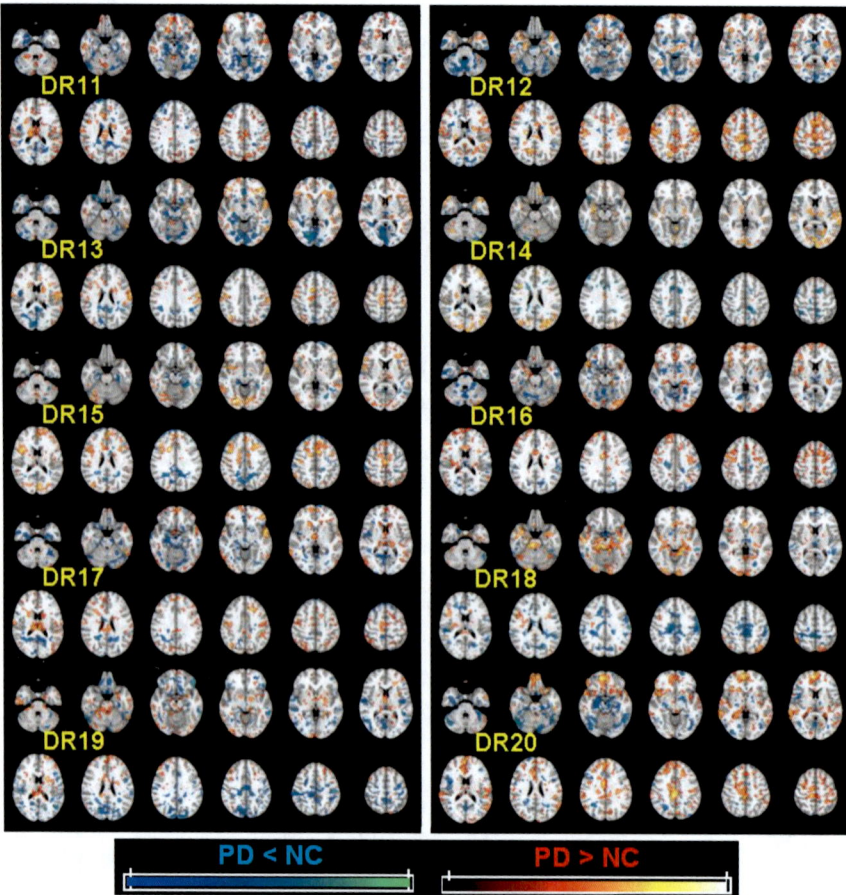

Figure 5. Statistical comparison map between PD and NC with $P < 0.01$ for the 11th-20th dual regression components (DR11-DR20). Red: PD > NC and Blue: PD < NC. Lower inter-connectivity in the basal ganglia, visual cortex, motor and supplementary cortex as well as cerebellum were found in PD patients in most of DR components compared to controls (such as in DR18 and DR19, blue color). Hyper-connectivity in the motor, supplementary motor and frontal networks with the most significant differences of DR12 and DR20 (thalamic and frontal networks respectively) were also demonstrated in PD compared to controls (red color).

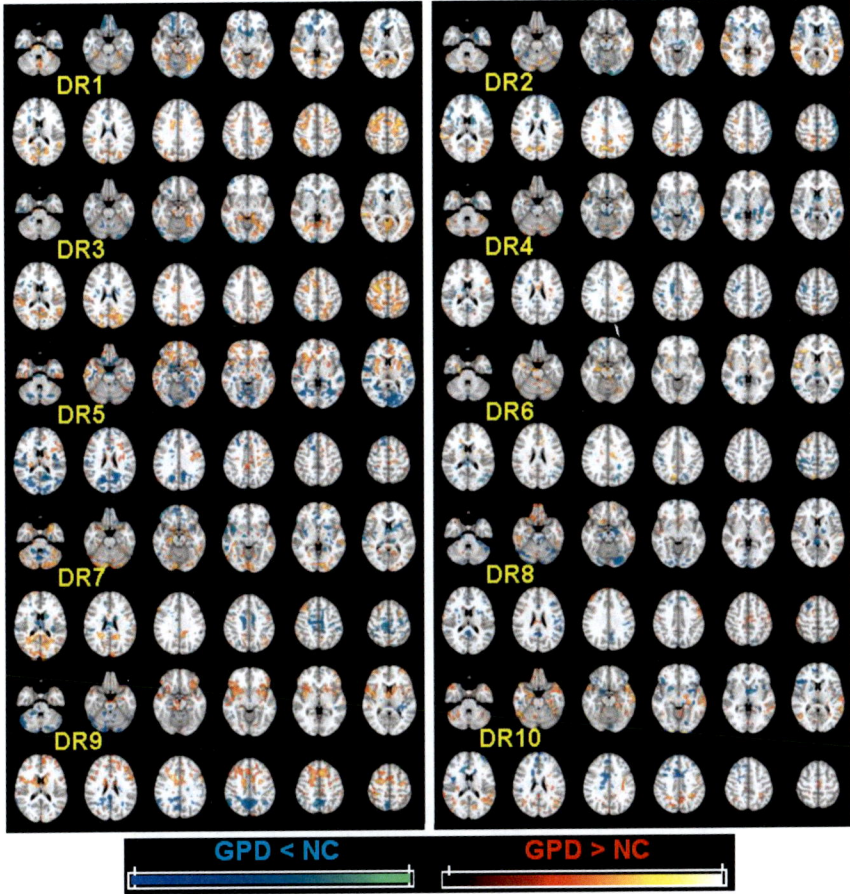

Figure 6. Statistical comparison map between GPD and NC with P < 0.01 for the first 1-10 dual regression components (DR1-DR10). Red: GPD > NC and Blue: GPD < NC.

However, higher inter-connectivity in the motor, supplementary motor and frontal networks with the most significant differences of DR12 and DR20 were also found in PD compared to controls (Figure 5 red color).

Statistical comparison map between GPD group and NC with P < 0.01 demonstrated similar results as to differences between PD and NC, with Figure 6 for the early ICA-DR 1st -10th components (DR1-DR10) comparisons and Figure 7 for the later 11th -20th DR components between GPD and NC. Finally, statistical comparison map with ICA-DR between prodromal (PM) group and NC with P < 0.01 demonstrated similar pattern but with slightly stronger or more hyper-connectivity results such as in the DAN, dorsolateral prefrontal cortex and motor/premotor areas, as to the differences between PD/GPD and NC groups.

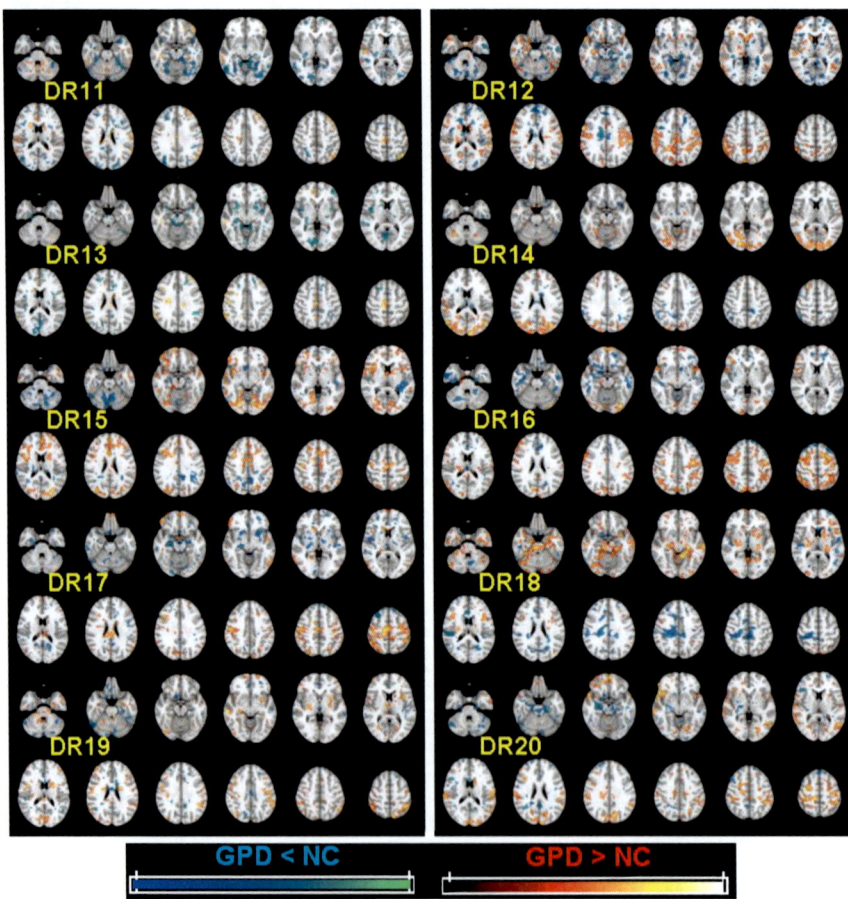

Figure 7. Statistical comparison map between GPD and NC with P < 0.01 for the 11th-20th dual regression components (DR11-DR20). Red: GPD > NC and Blue: GPD < NC.

Figure 8 illustrated the ICA-DR network comparisons of the early 10 components (DR1-DR10), and Figure 9 for the later 11-20th DR components between PM and NC groups. The basal ganglia showed relatively less hypo-connectivity in PM vs. NC compared to PD vs. NC, with decreased insular-DAN and putamen-mesolimbic but increased insular-DMN inter-network connectivities (such as in DR16 and DR20) were identified in PM/GPD compared to NC additionally.

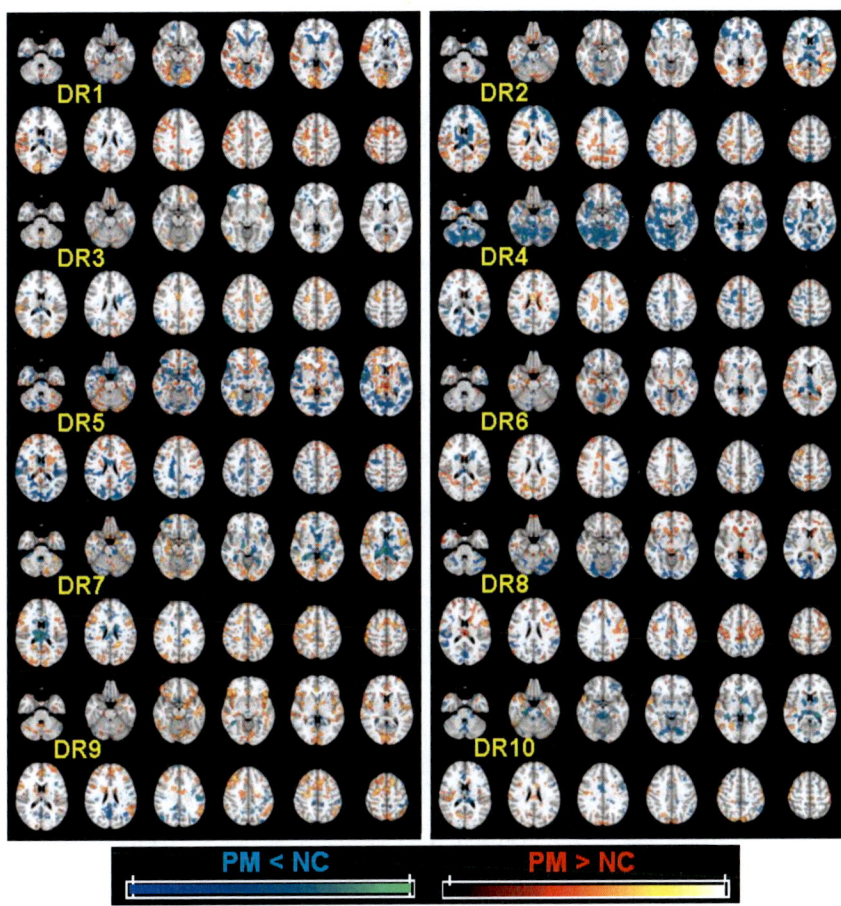

Figure 8. Statistical comparison map between PM and NC with P < 0.01 for the first 1-10 dual regression components (DR1-DR10). Red: PM > NC and Blue: PM < NC.

Furthermore, significant correlations between global VMHC and fALFF (a marker of neural activity) values in two groups of PD and NC and four groups of all participants were illustrated in Figure 10 respectively (both $r \geq 0.35$, $P \leq 0.04$). Also significant correlations existed between functional connectivity seeding from thalamic segment3 (occipital projection) and mean VMHC Z-value ($r = -0.72$, $P = 0.04$) (Figure 11).

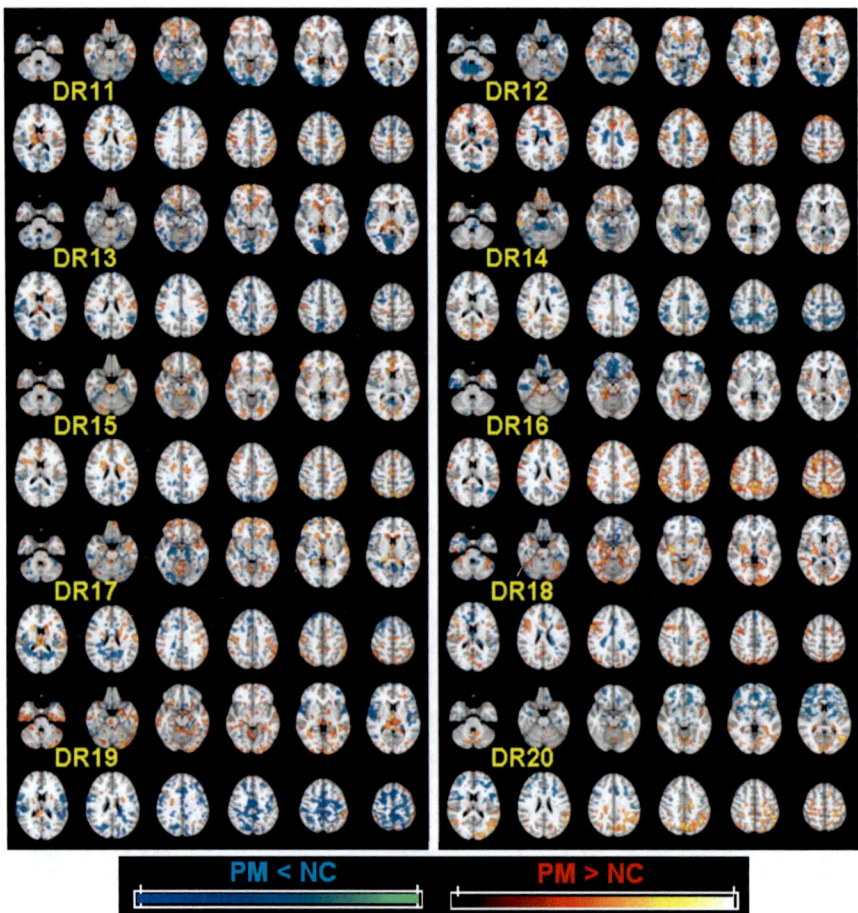

Figure 9. Statistical comparison map between PM and NC with P < 0.01 for the 11th-20th dual regression components (DR11-DR20). Red: PM > NC and Blue: PM < NC.

And strong correlations between caudate functional connectivity strength and global VMHC Z-value (r = 0.77, P = 0.03) was found in controls. A trend of correlation between middle temporal connectivity and VMHC, as well as between frontal eye field connectivity and VMHC were identified additionally (P < 0.1). In PD patients, stronger associations between putamen/ thalamic segment 4 (frontal projection) connectivities and global VMHC Z-value were found ($|r|\geq 0.54$, P ≤ 0.018), as well as between DMN connectivity and VMHC (P = 0.04). A trend existed between left thalamic connectivity and VMHC (P = 0.07) (Figure 12).

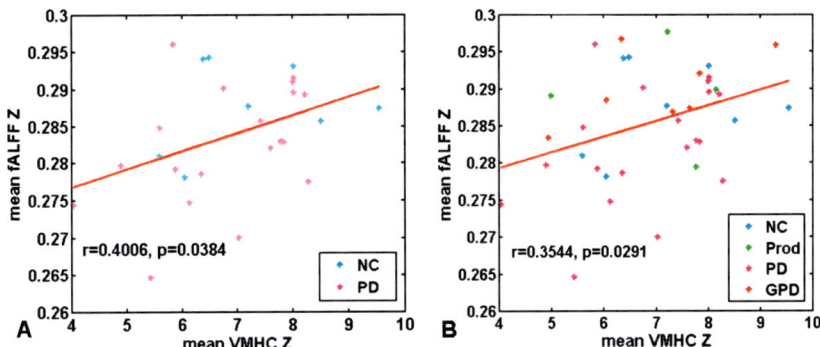

Figure 10. Significant correlations between global mean Z-values of VMHC and fALFF (a marker of neural activity) in two groups of PD and NC (A; r = 0.40, P = 0.04), and four groups including NC, PD, GPD and prodromal stage (Prod or PM) with all participants (B; r = 0.35, P = 0.03).

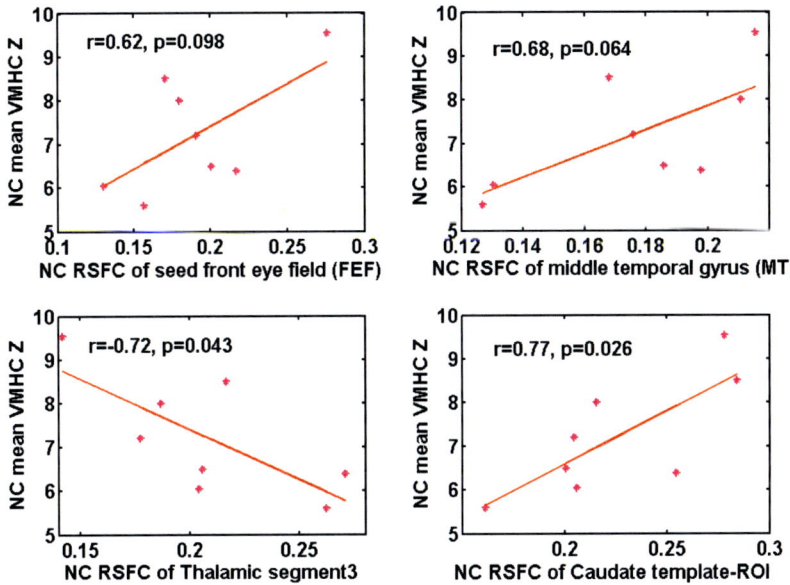

Figure 11. Correlations between global mean Z-values of VMHC and RSFC networks with conventional seeds in controls. Significant connections between global mean VMHC Z-value and RSFC seeding from thalamic segment3 (r = -0.72, P = 0.04) existed, as well as from caudate (r = 0.77, P = 0.03); also trends between VMHC and middle temporal/frontal eye field RSFC (r>0.61, P < 0.1).

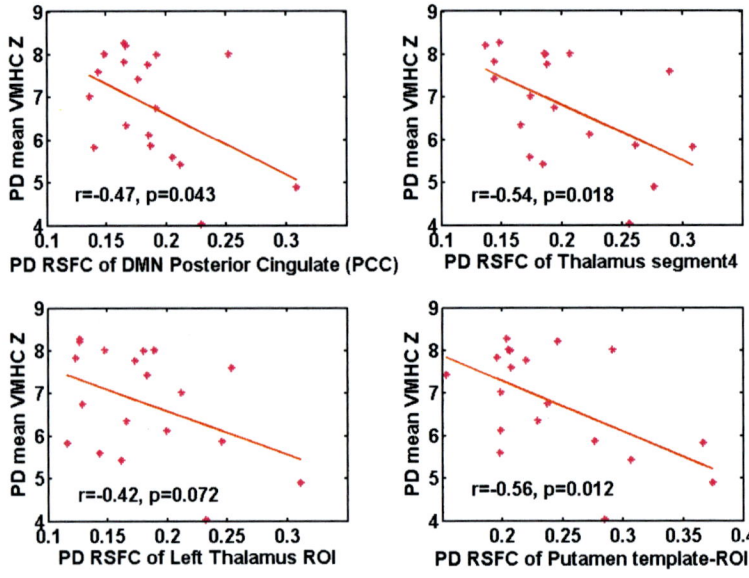

Figure 12. Correlations between global mean values of VMHC and RSFC in PD patients (A-D). Strong connections between putamen/ thalamic segment 4 connectivities and global VMHC Z-value in PD patients were found (right column; |r| ≥ 0.54, P ≤ 0.018), as well as between DMN connectivity and VMHC (P = 0.04). A trend existed between left thalamic connectivity and VMHC (P = 0.07).

With both measuring neural activity and connectivity, strong connections between RSFC and fALFF Z-values were present, in each group and more correlated in the control than PD group. For instance, in control group, significant correlations between fALFF and RSFC of thalamus (segments 1 and 5 for motor and premotor projections; $P < 0.005$), middle temporal gyrus ($P = 0.01$) and DMN ($P = 0.04$) were observed (Figure 13). In PD patients, only a marginal connection was found between fALFF and RSFC of dorsal medial prefrontal cortex (dMPFC) and thalamus (both $P = 0.05$) (Figure 14). Trends between global mean of fALFF and Z-values of RSFC of thalamic segment2 (sensory projection) / anterior medial prefrontal cortex (aMPFC) seeds were identified in addition (both $P = 0.08$). Less correlation between RSFC and fALFF in PD compared to NC was possibly due to the local injury reflected from fALFF and more dis-coordination or incoherence in PD patients.

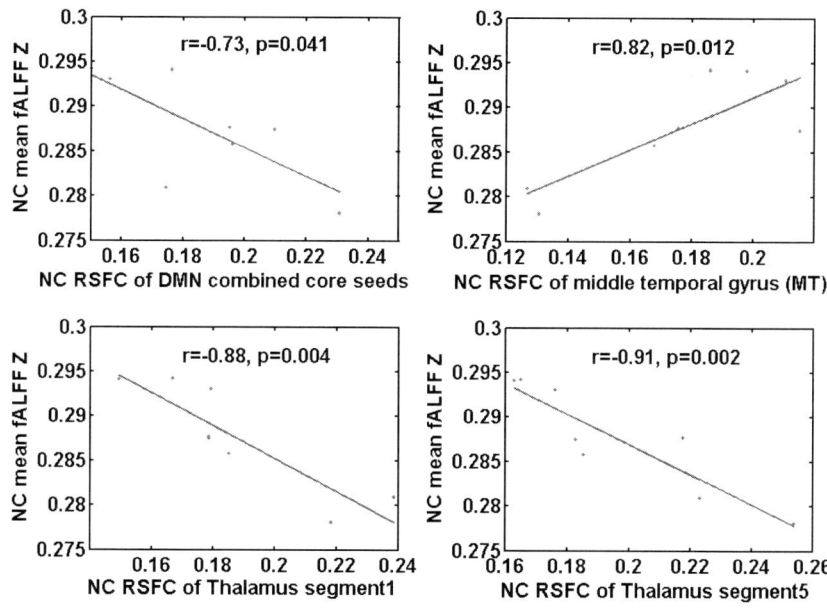

Figure 13. Significant correlations existed between global mean Z-values of fALFF and RSFC for control group in the thalamus (segments 4 and 5; r<-0.88, P < 0.005), middle temporal gyrus (r=0.82, P = 0.01) and DMN (r=-0.73, P = 0.04) (A-D). With both measuring neural activity and connectivity, strong connections between functional connectivity with RSFC and fALFF Z-values were present.

In addition, the amplitude at low frequency sub-band of slow wave S4 (0.027-0.073 Hz) and conventional fALFF at 0.01-0.08Hz band presented higher global mean value in the GPD group compared to PD group with P = 0.02 and P = 0.008 respectively (Figure 15). No other significant differences of fALFF global mean values or images between sub-groups were found (P > 0.05). Overall, small-worldness analysis based on fMRI connectivity data in NC and PD showed increased absolute local efficiency (CCFS) in PD for possible functional compensation with slightly decreased relative global efficiency (Lamda, λ, shortest path length) in PD patients compared to controls (Figure 16). Group mean values at each sparsity level across subjects in two groups were used for comparison. The overall small-worldness factor (Sigma, σ) presented relatively higher values in PD compared to NC, likely resulted from the higher local efficiency in patients (Figure 16B).

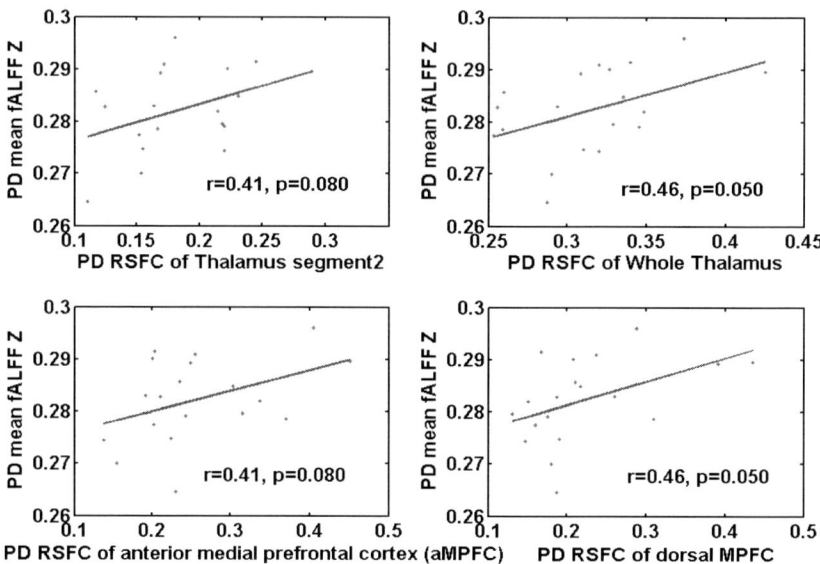

Figure 14. Correlations between global mean Z-values of fALFF and RSFC in PD patients (A-D). Only a marginal connection was found between fALFF and RSFC of dorsal medial prefrontal cortex (dMPFC) and thalamus (both P = 0.05). A trend between fALFF and RSFC of thalamic segment2 and anterior medial prefrontal cortex (aMPFC) was identified in addition (both P = 0.08).

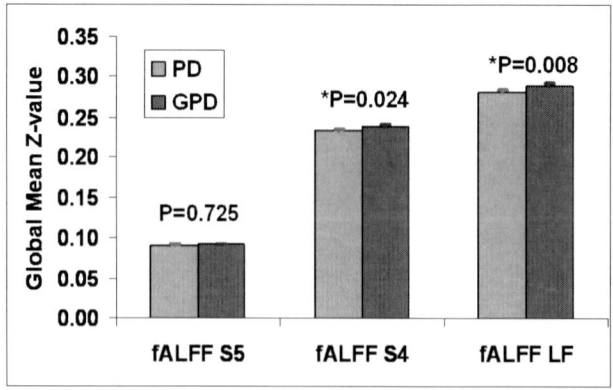

Figure 15. Significant fALFF differences between PD vs. GPD two groups at low frequency slow-waves of sub-band S4 (0.027-0.073 Hz; P = 0.024) and conventional low frequency (LF) band of 0.01-0.08Hz (P = 0.008), with higher global mean values of fALFF in GPD compared to PD.

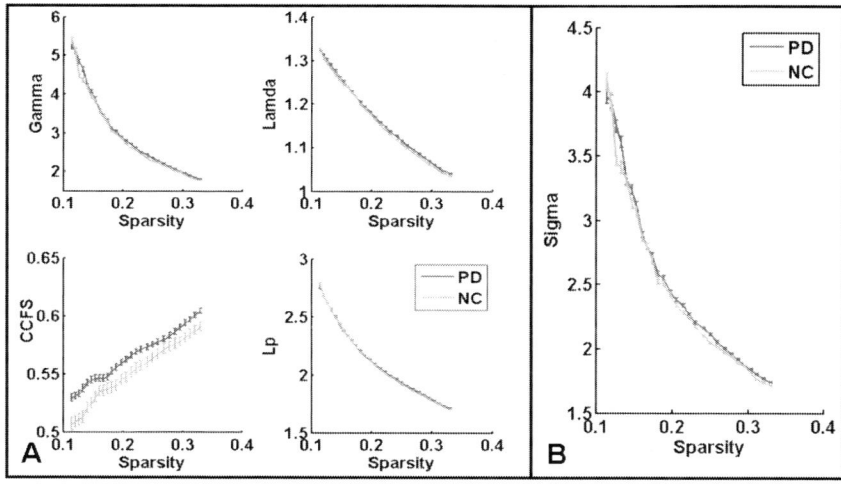

Figure 16. A: Small-worldness analysis based on fMRI connectivity data in NC and PD showing slightly decreased absolute global efficiency (Lamda, shortest path length) in PD (red dark line) compared to controls (blue light line), with the compensation of increased local relative efficiency (CCFS) in patients. B: Group mean values at each sparsity level across subjects in each of the two groups were used for comparison. The overall small-worldness factor (Sigma) presented relatively higher values in PD compared to NC.

Table 5. Classification results for four classifier evaluation: Accuracy of identifying each group using the VMHC metric with the maximum criterion; middle three columns for four groups classification (PD, GPD, PM and NC), while last column highlighted results of only two groups for identifying PD from NC

Maximal criterion of four classifiers	PD	GPD	PM	PD vs. NC (Inclusion of only two groups)
SVM + QP	0.6667	0.8333	0.8947	0.8462
SVM + RBF	0.6667	0.8333	0.8947	0.7692
KNN	0.6667	0.8333	0.8947	0.8462
SVM + Polynomial	0.7222	0.8333	0.8947	0.8462

Finally, classification results showed optimal accuracy of 0.90 in identifying PM from the rest of three groups (NC, PD and GPD) with the global mean Z-value of VMHC map, and 0.83 for GPD classification as well as 0.72 for PD classification with the maximum criterion (Table 5).

With only two groups (PD and NC) included for classification, three out of four classifiers reached accuracy of 0.85 for PD identification (last column in Table 5). And classifier SVM with polynomial kernel function obtained the best results among the four classifiers.

4. DISCUSSION

The swallow tail sign in SN as the imaging signature was mostly observed with significantly lower VMHC values comparing PD to NC; and some portion (especially posterior lateral session) was present in the VMHC difference image comparing GPD to NC together with small regions in the basal ganglia in PM and NC comparison. Lower VMHC in multiple other brain regions including cortical orbitofrontal and temporal cortices as well as subcortical striatum, hypothalamus and thalamus were also present in three patient groups including PD, GPD and PM compared to NC. Most of these regions with lower VMHC also had gray matter atrophy based on structural VBM results, such as inferior and middle temporal cortex, medial-orbito frontal cortex, dorsolateral prefrontal cortex, motor and supplementary motor cortices as well as small regions in the posterior basal ganglia, right insula and cerebellum. Gray matter atrophies in cortical frontal and temporal regions as well as SN and cerebellum had been confirmed by several studies, and were linked with impaired performance such as movement speed, accuracy, hallucination and cognitive memory dysfunction in PD patients [33-36]. The swallow tail sign signature in PD had further been validated with the DTI data that presented significantly lower FA in the right SN middle portion in PD patients compared to NC. The lower DTI FA values in SN (middle and caudal sessions) were also confirmed in other studies and had been applied in disease classification involving tremor in PD with acceptable accuracy [37-39]. Significant correlations were observed between VMHC and fALFF (a marker of neural activity) in two groups of PD and NC and four groups of all participants. These correlations implicated that the lower VMHC observed in PD/GPD patients might be due to the lower neural activity at local region in the SN in addition to the interhemispheric discoordination function of the SN, especially the swallow tail regions and the striatum that might affect the motor, learning and reward systems. Our results were in line with the lower myelin content reflected from VMHC that might be related to disease severity together with the abnormal intrinsic neural oscillations of slow-wave in the corticostriatal network affecting motor impairment, communication and perception in PD that were recently reported [40-42]. For instance, higher VMHC functional coordination in GPD patients compared to PD in clusters of orbitofrontal cortex, inferior temporal, superior parietal and occipital cortices were consistent with the fALFF findings of higher slow wave S4 within the low frequency band (i.e., more neuronal activity and abnormally higher coherence globally) as well as the larger conventional low frequency fluctuation in GPD group.

Moreover, several disrupted brain networks in PD compared to NC were identified with ICA-based DR remapping algorithm, such as basal ganglia and temporal/orbitofrontal circuits, DMN and thalamic network, FPN, motor and supplementary motor network, superior/medial frontal, temporal cortex and auditory networks. In contrast, a few other networks including inter-frontal and motor/supplementary motor, dorsolateral prefrontal and visual cortices also presented hyper-connectivity in the PD patients, possibly for functional compensation. GPD group and NC comparison demonstrated similar DR functional connectivity results as to differences between PD and NC, while prodromal (PM) group and NC comparison presented similar but slightly stronger (more positive or hyper-connectivity) results as to differences between PD/GPD and NC. The hyper-connectivity patterns such as in the dorsolateral prefrontal and supplementary motor networks in PM patients were mainly for compensation and protection mechanisms with the possible maximal brain functional output in the transitional stage. Less insular-DAN but more insular-DMN inter-network connectivity patterns were exhibited in PM/GPD compared to NC groups, probably relating to attentional deficit and misperception behavior in patients [13, 16-17].

Additionally as expected, the UPDRS motor score was significantly higher in PD and GPD groups compared to controls. Moreover, higher frame displacement (FD) due to abrupt motion artifact was detected in the RS-fMRI data of PD patients compared to controls, especially from the mean top quartile and decile portions. Both higher UPDRS and FD values in PD/GPD suggested that movement disorder such as tremor in PD patients might be the reason of motion artifacts during image acquisition. There was no significant difference between prodromal patients and NC for both UPDRS and FD scores, possibly due to the smaller number of participants in this group. The typical basal ganglia network disruption to Parkinsonism including tremor and slowness, corticostriatal and prefrontal connectivity impact on impulsivity control, reward seeking and accuracy, frontal and temporal inter-network influence on memory, emotion and executive function had been validated with several recent works [43-45]. Our ICA-DR network connectivity results also had the advantage to reveal the complex intra- and inter-connections of multiple brain circuits that might be disrupted in PD, including the within- and between-modulation of DMN, DAN and FPN, motor-sensory circuit together with the insular-auditory salience and thalamocortical networks for timely and coherent brain status switching, communication, planning and execution [27, 46, 47]. The hyper-connectivity pattern from the motor/premotor areas and DAN might serve as the compensation role and could also lead to dysfunction such as altered motor behavior, impaired executive function as well as loss of mutual inhibition and systematic coordination among brain networks when disease progresses [48, 49].

Furthermore, positive correlation between VMHC and RSFC seeded from the caudate-frontal region and negative association between VMHC and thalamic segment3 (occipital projection) RSFC in controls were observed. While in PD patients, significantly negative correlations between VMHC and RSFC seeded from the DMN posterior cingulate, putamen as well as thalamic segment 4 (temporal projection) were found ($P < 0.05$). Some RSFC networks in the thalamus and DMN regions were also connected to the fALFF values with both measuring low-frequency activity and connectivity and stronger in control groups, possible due to local neuronal injury in patients. These correlational results between global VMHC and RSFC values were consistent with the differences found with each voxel-wise imaging metric separately, such as both lower VMHC and intra-network functional connectivity in the DMN, putamen-mesolimbic and thalamo-cortical networks in PD/GPD patients. Moreover, classification based on single global VMHC z-value could achieve accuracy of 0.90/0.83/0.72 for identifying PM/GPD/PD from the rest of other three groups. And accuracy reached 0.85 with 5-fold cross-validation for classifying PD from NC when including only these two groups based on global VMHC. Our results confirmed the deficits of interhemispheric coordination and functional connectivity (pathway dysconnectivity) as well as possible local neuronal activity injury in PD/GPD patients from multiple brain networks such as DMN, FPN and thalamus, in addition to the basal ganglia dysfunction [50].

Since there were several hyper-connectivity regions such as motor and visual networks in PD, the global efficiency was slightly lower in patients together with higher local efficiency based on brain network integration analysis. Reduction of global efficiency in PD had been previously reported with fMRI data and confirmed with the microstructural DTI findings, that might be used to monitor treatment efficacy [51-53]. Identifying presymptomatic individuals with early prevention, developing new multiomic biomarkers related to oxidative stress, protein aggregation and inflammation risk factors in addition to applications of more advanced imaging technique such as better SN segmentation and inter-module longitudinal analysis will be some future works [54-56].

In summary, both functional VMHC/ICA-DR and structural DTI results revealed the swallow tail sign signature in PD/GPD patients compared to NC. Furthermore, the lower VMHC regions co-localized with the gray matter atrophy regions in patients, including inferior and middle temporal cortex, lingual, medial-orbito frontal cortex, dorsolateral prefrontal cortex, motor and supplementary motor cortices, striatum, as well as small regions in the posterior basal ganglia, right insular and cerebellum. Reduced functional connectivity of multiple brain circuits in PD/GPD/PM compared to NC were identified with ICA-DR method including basal ganglia and temporal/orbitofrontal circuits, default mode and thalamo-cortical networks, FPN, motor and supplementary motor networks, superior/medial frontal, temporal cortex and auditory networks, probably resulted from both intra- and inter-network functional discoordination in patients. Network rerouting including hyper-connectivity in the motor, supplementary motor and dorsolateral prefrontal and visual cortices were also present in these patients for possible functional compensation. And global efficiency based on functional connectivity was lower in patients with slightly higher local efficiency. Furthermore, global VMHC correlated with global fALFF and functional connectivity in the DMN and thalamus/putamen network. Quantitative MRI-based VMHC and ICA-DR algorithms had been validated to be unique conductivity and coordination imaging biomarkers for PD with precise identification of disease abnormalities and high correlations with other quantitative metrics as well as acceptable accuracy for classifying patients.

Acknowledgments

Data collection and sharing for this project was funded by the Alzheimer's Disease Neuroimaging Initiative (ADNI) (National Institutes of Health Grant U01 AG024904) and DOD ADNI (Department of Defense award number W81XWH-12-2-0012). ADNI is funded by the National Institute on Aging, the National Institute of Biomedical Imaging and Bioengineering, and through generous contributions from the following: AbbVie, Alzheimer's Association; Alzheimer's Drug Discovery Foundation; Araclon Biotech; BioClinica, Inc.; Biogen; Bristol-Myers Squibb Company; CereSpir, Inc.; Cogstate; Eisai Inc.; Elan Pharmaceuticals, Inc.; Eli Lilly and Company; EuroImmun; F. Hoffmann-La Roche Ltd and its affiliated company Genentech, Inc.; Fujirebio; GE Healthcare; IXICO Ltd.; Janssen Alzheimer Immunotherapy Research and Development, LLC.; Johnson and Johnson Pharmaceutical Research and Development LLC.; Lumosity; Lundbeck; Merck and Co., Inc.; Meso Scale Diagnostics, LLC.; NeuroRx Research; Neurotrack Technologies;

Novartis Pharmaceuticals Corporation; Pfizer Inc.; Piramal Imaging; Servier; Takeda Pharmaceutical Company; and Transition Therapeutics. The Canadian Institutes of Health Research is providing funds to support ADNI clinical sites in Canada. Private sector contributions are facilitated by the Foundation for the National Institutes of Health (www.fnih.org). The grantee organization is the Northern California Institute for Research and Education, and the study is coordinated by the Alzheimer's Therapeutic Research Institute at the University of Southern California. ADNI data are disseminated by the Laboratory for NeuroImaging at the University of Southern California.

Data used in preparation of this article were obtained from the Alzheimer's Disease Neuroimaging Initiative (ADNI) database website (adni.loni.usc.edu). The author is one of the investigators of ADNI data cohort. The other investigators within the ADNI might contribute to the design and implementation of ADNI and/or provide data but did not participate in analysis or writing of this report.

REFERENCES

[1] Zeighami Y, Ulla M, Iturria-Medina Y, Dadar M, Zhang Y, Larcher KM, Fonov V, Evans AC, Collins DL, Dagher A. Network structure of brain atrophy in de novo Parkinson's disease. *Elife*. 2015 Sep 7;4:e08440. doi: 10.7554/eLife.08440. PMID: 26344547; PMCID: PMC4596689.

[2] Zeighami Y, Fereshtehnejad SM, Dadar M, Collins DL, Postuma RB, Mišić B, Dagher A. A clinical-anatomical signature of Parkinson's disease identified with partial least squares and magnetic resonance imaging. *Neuroimage*. 2019 Apr 15;190:69-78. doi: 10.1016/j.neuroimage.2017.12.050. Epub 2017 Dec 19. PMID: 29277406.

[3] Cheng Z, Zhang J, He N, Li Y, Wen Y, Xu H, Tang R, Jin Z, Haacke EM, Yan F, Qian D. Radiomic Features of the Nigrosome-1 Region of the Substantia Nigra: Using Quantitative Susceptibility Mapping

to Assist the Diagnosis of Idiopathic Parkinson's Disease. *Front Aging Neurosci.* 2019 Jul 16;11:167. doi: 10.3389/fnagi.2019.00167.

[4] Niethammer M, Feigin A, Eidelberg D. Functional neuroimaging in Parkinson's disease. *Cold Spring Harb Perspect Med.* 2012 May; 2(5):a009274. doi: 10.1101/cshperspect.a009274. PMID: 22553499; PMCID: PMC3331691.

[5] Rolinski M, Griffanti L, Piccini P, Roussakis AA, Szewczyk-Krolikowski K, Menke RA, Quinnell T, Zaiwalla Z, Klein JC, Mackay CE, Hu MT. Basal ganglia dysfunction in idiopathic REM sleep behaviour disorder parallels that in early Parkinson's disease. *Brain.* 2016 Aug;139(Pt 8):2224-34. doi: 10.1093/brain/aww124. Epub 2016 Jun 12. PMID: 27297241; PMCID: PMC4958897.

[6] Peraza LR, Nesbitt D, Lawson RA, Duncan GW, Yarnall AJ, Khoo TK, Kaiser M, Firbank MJ, O'Brien JT, Barker RA, Brooks DJ, Burn DJ, Taylor JP. Intra- and inter-network functional alterations in Parkinson's disease with mild cognitive impairment. *Hum Brain Mapp.* 2017 Mar;38(3):1702-1715. doi: 10.1002/hbm.23499. Epub 2017 Jan 13. PMID: 28084651; PMCID: PMC6866883.

[7] Wu T, Ma Y, Zheng Z, Peng S, Wu X, Eidelberg D, Chan P. Parkinson's disease-related spatial covariance pattern identified with resting-state functional MRI. *J Cereb Blood Flow Metab.* 2015 Nov;35(11):1764-70. doi: 10.1038/jcbfm.2015.118. Epub 2015 Jun 3. PMID: 26036935; PMCID: PMC4635231.

[8] Wu T, Wang J, Wang C, Hallett M, Zang Y, Wu X, Chan P. Basal ganglia circuits changes in Parkinson's disease patients. *Neurosci Lett.* 2012 Aug 22;524(1):55-9. doi: 10.1016/j.neulet.2012.07.012. Epub 2012 Jul 17. PMID: 22813979; PMCID: PMC4163196.

[9] Badea L, Onu M, Wu T, Roceanu A, Bajenaru O. Exploring the reproducibility of functional connectivity alterations in Parkinson's disease. *PLoS One.* 2017 Nov 28;12(11):e0188196. doi: 10.1371/journal.pone.0188196. Erratum in: PLoS One. 2018 May 3;13(5):e0197121. PMID: 29182621; PMCID: PMC5705108.

[10] Vo A, Sako W, Fujita K, Peng S, Mattis PJ, Skidmore FM, Ma Y, Uluğ AM, Eidelberg D. Parkinson's disease-related network

topographies characterized with resting state functional MRI. *Hum Brain Mapp.* 2017 Feb;38(2):617-630. doi: 10.1002/hbm.23260. Epub 2016 May 21. PMID: 27207613; PMCID: PMC5118197.

[11] Tessitore A, Giordano A, De Micco R, Russo A, Tedeschi G. Sensorimotor connectivity in Parkinson's disease: the role of functional neuroimaging. *Front Neurol.* 2014 Sep 24;5:180. doi: 10.3389/fneur.2014.00180. PMID: 25309505; PMCID: PMC 4173645.

[12] Boon LI, Hepp DH, Douw L, van Geenen N, Broeders TAA, Geurts JJG, Berendse HW, Schoonheim MM. Functional connectivity between resting-state networks reflects decline in executive function in Parkinson's disease: A longitudinal fMRI study. *Neuroimage Clin.* 2020;28:102468. doi: 10.1016/j.nicl.2020.102468. Epub 2020 Oct 15. PMID: 33383608; PMCID: PMC7581965.

[13] Shine JM, Halliday GM, Gilat M, Matar E, Bolitho SJ, Carlos M, Naismith SL, Lewis SJ. The role of dysfunctional attentional control networks in visual misperceptions in Parkinson's disease. *Hum Brain Mapp.* 2014 May;35(5):2206-19. doi: 10.1002/hbm. 22321. Epub 2013 Jun 13. PMID: 23760982; PMCID: PMC6869072.

[14] Valsasina P, Hidalgo de la Cruz M, Filippi M, Rocca MA. Characterizing Rapid Fluctuations of Resting State Functional Connectivity in Demyelinating, Neurodegenerative, and Psychiatric Conditions: From Static to Time-Varying Analysis. *Front Neurosci.* 2019 Jul 10;13:618. doi: 10.3389/fnins.2019.00618. PMID: 31354402; PMCID: PMC6636554.

[15] Zhu H, Huang J, Deng L, He N, Cheng L, Shu P, Yan F, Tong S, Sun J, Ling H. Abnormal Dynamic Functional Connectivity Associated With Subcortical Networks in Parkinson's Disease: A Temporal Variability Perspective. *Front Neurosci.* 2019 Feb 19;13:80. doi: 10.3389/fnins.2019.00080. PMID: 30837825; PMCID: PMC6389716.

[16] Miloserdov K, Schmidt-Samoa C, Williams K, Weinrich CA, Kagan I, Bürk K, Trenkwalder C, Bähr M, Wilke M. Aberrant functional connectivity of resting state networks related to misperceptions and

intra-individual variability in Parkinson's disease. *Neuroimage Clin.* 2020;25:102076. doi: 10.1016/j.nicl.2019.102076. Epub 2019 Nov 5. PMID: 31794926; PMCID: PMC6906716.

[17] Madhyastha TM, Askren MK, Zhang J, Leverenz JB, Montine TJ, Grabowski TJ. Group comparison of spatiotemporal dynamics of intrinsic networks in Parkinson's disease. *Brain.* 2015 Sep;138(Pt 9):2672-86. doi: 10.1093/brain/awv189. Epub 2015 Jul 14. PMID: 26173859; PMCID: PMC4643623.

[18] Rubbert C, Mathys C, Jockwitz C, Hartmann CJ, Eickhoff SB, Hoffstaedter F, Caspers S, Eickhoff CR, Sigl B, Teichert NA, Südmeyer M, Turowski B, Schnitzler A, Caspers J. Machine-learning identifies Parkinson's disease patients based on resting-state between-network functional connectivity. *Br J Radiol.* 2019 Sep; 92(1101):20180886. doi: 10.1259/bjr.20180886. Epub 2019 May 14. PMID: 30994036; PMCID: PMC6732922.

[19] Tessitore A, Cirillo M, De Micco R. Functional Connectivity Signatures of Parkinson's Disease. *J Parkinsons Dis.* 2019;9(4):637-652. doi: 10.3233/JPD-191592. PMID: 31450512; PMCID: PMC 6839494.

[20] Nackaerts E, D'Cruz N, Dijkstra BW, Gilat M, Kramer T, Nieuwboer A. Towards understanding neural network signatures of motor skill learning in Parkinson's disease and healthy aging. *Br J Radiol.* 2019 Sep;92(1101):20190071. doi: 10.1259/bjr.20190071. Epub 2019 May 14. PMID: 30982328; PMCID: PMC6732914.

[21] Saeed U, Lang AE, Masellis M. Neuroimaging Advances in Parkinson's Disease and Atypical Parkinsonian Syndromes. *Front Neurol.* 2020 Oct 15;11:572976. doi: 10.3389/fneur.2020.572976. PMID: 33178113; PMCID: PMC7593544.

[22] Zhou Y, Milham MP, Lui YW, Miles L, Reaume J, Sodickson DK, Grossman RI, Ge Y. Default-mode network disruption in mild traumatic brain injury. *Radiology.* 2012 Dec;265(3):882-92. doi: 10.1148/radiol.12120748. PMID: 23175546; PMCID: PMC3504316.

[23] Zhou Y, Milham M, Zuo XN, Kelly C, Jaggi H, Herbert J, Grossman RI, Ge Y. Functional homotopic changes in multiple sclerosis with

resting-state functional MR imaging. *AJNR Am J Neuroradiol.* 2013 Jun-Jul;34(6):1180-7. doi: 10.3174/ajnr.A3386. Epub 2013 Jan 24. PMID: 23348760; PMCID: PMC3707620.

[24] Zhou Y. *Multiparametric Imaging in Neurodegenerative Disease.* Nova Publishers. 2020.

[25] Zhou Y. *Neuroimaging in Multiple Sclerosis.* Nova Science Publishers. 2017a.

[26] Zhou Y. *Functional Neuroimaging with Multiple Modalities: Principle, Device and Applicaitons.* Nova Science Publishers. 2016.

[27] Zhou Y, Lui YW, Zuo XN, Milham MP, Reaume J, Grossman RI, Ge Y. Characterization of thalamo-cortical association using amplitude and connectivity of functional MRI in mild traumatic brain injury. *J Magn Reson Imaging.* 2014 Jun;39(6):1558-68. doi: 10.1002/jmri.24310. Epub 2013 Sep 6. PMID: 24014176; PMCID: PMC3872273.

[28] Zuo XN, Kelly C, Adelstein JS, Klein DF, Castellanos FX, Milham MP. Reliable intrinsic connectivity networks: test-retest evaluation using ICA and dual regression approach. *Neuroimage.* 2010 Feb 1;49(3):2163-77. doi: 10.1016/j.neuroimage. 2009.10.080. Epub 2009 Nov 5. PMID: 19896537; PMCID: PMC2877508.

[29] Zhou Y. Small world properties changes in mild traumatic brain injury. *J Magn Reson Imaging.* 2017 Aug;46(2):518-527. doi: 10.1002/jmri.25548. Epub 2016 Nov 30. PMID: 27902865; PMCID: PMC5449268.

[30] Zhou Y. *Neuroimaging in Mild Traumatic Brain Injury.* Nova Science Publishers. 2017b.

[31] Zhou Y. *Mild Cognitive Impairment (MCI): Diagnosis, Prevalence and Quality of Life.* Nova Science Publishers 2017 Chapter 1;1-46.

[32] Zhou Y. *Imaging and Multiomic Biomarker Applications: Advances in Early Alzheimer's Disease.* Nova Science Publishers. 2021.

[33] Xu X, Han Q, Lin J, Wang L, Wu F, Shang H. Grey matter abnormalities in Parkinson's disease: a voxel-wise meta-analysis. *Eur J Neurol.* 2020 Apr;27(4):653-659. doi: 10.1111/ene.14132. Epub 2019 Dec 23. PMID: 31770481.

[34] Gao Y, Nie K, Huang B, Mei M, Guo M, Xie S, Huang Z, Wang L, Zhao J, Zhang Y, Wang L. Changes of brain structure in Parkinson's disease patients with mild cognitive impairment analyzed via VBM technology. *Neurosci Lett.* 2017 Sep 29;658:121-132. doi: 10.1016/j.neulet.2017.08.028. Epub 2017 Aug 18. PMID: 28823894.

[35] Donzuso G, Monastero R, Cicero CE, Luca A, Mostile G, Giuliano L, Baschi R, Caccamo M, Gagliardo C, Palmucci S, Zappia M, Nicoletti A. Neuroanatomical changes in early Parkinson's disease with mild cognitive impairment: a VBM study; the Parkinson's Disease Cognitive Impairment Study (PaCoS). *Neurol Sci.* 2021 Jan 14. doi: 10.1007/s10072-020-05034-9. Epub ahead of print. PMID: 33447925.

[36] Lawn T, Ffytche D. Cerebellar correlates of visual hallucinations in Parkinson's disease and Charles Bonnet Syndrome. *Cortex.* 2021 Feb;135:311-325. doi: 10.1016/j.cortex.2020.10.024. Epub 2020 Dec 5. PMID: 33390262.

[37] Vaillancourt DE, Spraker MB, Prodoehl J, Abraham I, Corcos DM, Zhou XJ, Comella CL, Little DM. High-resolution diffusion tensor imaging in the substantia nigra of de novo Parkinson disease. *Neurology.* 2009 Apr 21;72(16):1378-84. doi: 10.1212/01.wnl. 0000340982.01727.6e. Epub 2009 Jan 7. Erratum in: Neurology. 2009 Jun 9;72(23):2059. PMID: 19129507; PMCID: PMC2677508.

[38] Prodoehl J, Li H, Planetta PJ, Goetz CG, Shannon KM, Tangonan R, Comella CL, Simuni T, Zhou XJ, Leurgans S, Corcos DM, Vaillancourt DE. Diffusion tensor imaging of Parkinson's disease, atypical Parkinsonism, and essential tremor. *Mov Disord.* 2013 Nov;28(13):1816-22. doi: 10.1002/mds.25491. Epub 2013 May 14. PMID: 23674400; PMCID: PMC3748146.

[39] Atkinson-Clement C, Pinto S, Eusebio A, Coulon O. Diffusion tensor imaging in Parkinson's disease: Review and meta-analysis. *Neuroimage Clin.* 2017 Jul 15;16:98-110. doi: 10.1016/j.nicl.2017. 07.011. PMID: 28765809; PMCID: PMC5527156.

[40] Dean DC 3rd, Sojkova J, Hurley S, Kecskemeti S, Okonkwo O, Bendlin BB, Theisen F, Johnson SC, Alexander AL, Gallagher CL.

Alterations of Myelin Content in Parkinson's Disease: A Cross-Sectional Neuroimaging Study. *PLoS One.* 2016 Oct 5;11(10): e0163774. doi: 10.1371/journal.pone.0163774. PMID: 27706215; PMCID: PMC5051727.

[41] Guan X, Guo T, Zeng Q, Wang J, Zhou C, Liu C, Wei H, Zhang Y, Xuan M, Gu Q, Xu X, Huang P, Pu J, Zhang B, Zhang MM. Oscillation-specific nodal alterations in early to middle stages Parkinson's disease. *Transl Neurodegener.* 2019 Nov 15;8:36. doi: 10.1186/s40035-019-0177-5. PMID: 31807287; PMCID: PMC6857 322.

[42] Zhang J, Wei L, Hu X, Zhang Y, Zhou D, Li C, Wang X, Feng H, Yin X, Xie B, Wang J. Specific frequency band of amplitude low-frequency fluctuation predicts Parkinson's disease. *Behav Brain Res.* 2013 Sep 1;252:18-23. doi: 10.1016/j.bbr.2013.05.039. Epub 2013 May 29. PMID: 23727173.

[43] Szewczyk-Krolikowski K, Menke RA, Rolinski M, Duff E, Salimi-Khorshidi G, Filippini N, Zamboni G, Hu MT, Mackay CE. Functional connectivity in the basal ganglia network differentiates PD patients from controls. *Neurology.* 2014 Jul 15;83(3):208-14. doi: 10.1212/WNL.0000000000000592. Epub 2014 Jun 11. PMID: 24920856; PMCID: PMC4117363.

[44] Aracil-Bolaños I, Strafella AP. Molecular imaging and neural networks in impulse control disorders in Parkinson's disease. *Parkinsonism Relat Disord.* 2016 Jan;22 Suppl 1(Suppl 1):S101-5. doi: 10.1016/j.parkreldis.2015.08.003. Epub 2015 Aug 12. PMID: 26298389; PMCID: PMC4874782.

[45] Abós A, Baggio HC, Segura B, García-Díaz AI, Compta Y, Martí MJ, Valldeoriola F, Junqué C. Discriminating cognitive status in Parkinson's disease through functional connectomics and machine learning. *Sci Rep.* 2017 Mar 28;7:45347. doi: 10.1038/srep45347. PMID: 28349948; PMCID: PMC5368610.

[46] Baggio HC, Segura B, Junque C. Resting-state functional brain networks in Parkinson's disease. *CNS Neurosci Ther.* 2015

Oct;21(10):793-801. doi: 10.1111/cns.12417. Epub 2015 Jul 30. PMID: 26224057; PMCID: PMC6093256

[47] Lanskey JH, McColgan P, Schrag AE, Acosta-Cabronero J, Rees G, Morris HR, Weil RS. Can neuroimaging predict dementia in Parkinson's disease? *Brain.* 2018 Sep 1;141(9):2545-2560. doi: 10.1093/brain/awy211. PMID: 30137209; PMCID: PMC6113860.

[48] Lebedev AV, Westman E, Simmons A, Lebedeva A, Siepel FJ, Pereira JB, Aarsland D. Large-scale resting state network correlates of cognitive impairment in Parkinson's disease and related dopaminergic deficits. *Front Syst Neurosci.* 2014 Apr 3;8:45. doi: 10.3389/fnsys.2014.00045. PMID: 24765065; PMCID: PMC398 2053.

[49] Göttlich M, Münte TF, Heldmann M, Kasten M, Hagenah J, Krämer UM. Altered resting state brain networks in Parkinson's disease. *PLoS One.* 2013 Oct 28;8(10):e77336. doi: 10.1371/journal.pone.0077336. PMID: 24204812; PMCID: PMC3810472.

[50] Baggio HC, Sala-Llonch R, Segura B, Marti MJ, Valldeoriola F, Compta Y, Tolosa E, Junqué C. Functional brain networks and cognitive deficits in Parkinson's disease. *Hum Brain Mapp.* 2014 Sep;35(9):4620-34. doi: 10.1002/hbm.22499. Epub 2014 Mar 17. PMID: 24639411; PMCID: PMC6869398.

[51] Skidmore F, Korenkevych D, Liu Y, He G, Bullmore E, Pardalos PM. Connectivity brain networks based on wavelet correlation analysis in Parkinson fMRI data. *Neurosci Lett.* 2011 Jul 15;499(1):47-51. doi: 10.1016/j.neulet.2011.05.030. Epub 2011 May 23. PMID: 21624430.

[52] Vancea R, Simonyan K, Petracca M, Brys M, Di Rocco A, Ghilardi MF, Inglese M. Cognitive performance in mid-stage Parkinson's disease: functional connectivity under chronic antiparkinson treatment. *Brain Imaging Behav.* 2019 Feb;13(1):200-209. doi: 10.1007/s11682-017-9765-0. PMID: 28942477; PMCID: PMC5 866203.

[53] Gou L, Zhang W, Li C, Shi X, Zhou Z, Zhong W, Chen T, Wu X, Yang C, Guo D. Structural Brain Network Alteration and its

Correlation With Structural Impairments in Patients With Depression in de novo and Drug-Naïve Parkinson's Disease. *Front Neurol.* 2018 Jul 26;9:608. doi: 10.3389/fneur.2018.00608. PMID: 30093879.

[54] Perlmutter JS, Norris SA. Neuroimaging biomarkers for Parkinson disease: facts and fantasy. *Ann Neurol.* 2014 Dec;76(6):769-83. doi: 10.1002/ana.24291. Epub 2014 Nov 7. PMID: 25363872; PMCID: PMC4245400.

[55] Ren R, Sun Y, Zhao X, Pu X. Recent advances in biomarkers for Parkinson's disease focusing on biochemicals, omics and neuroimaging. *Clin Chem Lab Med.* 2015 Sep 1;53(10):1495-506. doi: 10.1515/cclm-2014-0783. PMID: 25581757.

[56] Manjón JV, Bertó A, Romero JE, Lanuza E, Vivo-Hernando R, Aparici-Robles F, Coupe P. pBrain: A novel pipeline for Parkinson related brain structure segmentation. *Neuroimage Clin.* 2020; 25:102184. doi: 10.1016/j.nicl.2020.102184. Epub 2020 Jan 15. PMID: 31982678; PMCID: PMC6992999.

Chapter 2

MOLECULAR IMAGING IN PARKINSON'S DISEASE AND PET/MRI APPLICATIONS

ABSTRACT

In addition to the previous MRI results of PD/GPD/PM in chapter 1, the purpose of Section 1 in this chapter is to reveal the PET molecular imaging abnormalities in these patients, including the dopamine transporter (DAT) and striatal binding ratio (SBR) data, as well as the vesicular monoamine transporter type 2 (VMAT2) with region-of interest (ROI) based quantifications. Expected lower SBR and DAT levels in PD compared to NC were found in the striatal caudate and putamen regions. Generally less VMAT2 densities in PD/GPD compared to NC were found in the bilateral mesial temporal cortex, caudate, orbitofrontal cortex, left frontal and occipital cortices, however with a lower level in PM compared to other groups were observed additionally. The PET molecular imaging results, showing reduced dopamine transporter and binding potential levels in striatum and less cortical (spare of parietal lobe) and caudate dopamine storage and pathway deficits, were in line with the MRI imaging results including swallow tail sign (dopaminergic neuron reductions in nigrosome-1 territory) in substantia nigra with less microstructural connectivity or conductivity, gray matter atrophy and lower interhemispheric coordination/functional connectivity in the cortical inferior/middle temporal and medial-orbito frontal regions.

Section II reviewed the multimodal PET/MRI applications in brain science and neurological diseases, and further elucidated PET/MRI combination for revealing the imaging differences affected with multiple physiological and neuropathological mechanisms. The representative example demonstrated the multiparametric quantification with the integrated PET/MRI imaging for the biological factor characterization.

Keywords: Parkinson's disease, dopamine, swallow tail sign, dopamine transporter, striatal binding ratio, vesicular monoamine transporter, caudate, putamen, substantia nigra, PET/MRI, multimodal integration, multiparametric quantification, disease mechanism, gender differences, biological factor characterization

1. MOLECULAR IMAGING IN PARKINSON'S DEMENTIA

1.1. Introduction

Parkinson's disease (PD) is the second most common neurodegenerative disorder, with overall of 0.2% prevalence rate; affecting 0.5-1% individuals aged 65-69 years old, and 1-3% for 80+ elderly people. The typical signs include tremor, slowness of movement and rigidity; with occasionally neuropsychiatric problems such as depression, anxiety and apathy [1, 2]. In brain, the substantia nigra (SN) is the earliest affected brain region causing decreased dopamine transmitter, with possible basal ganglia-thalamo-cortical motor and other cognitive circuits involved. Symptomatic and atypical Parkinsonism syndrome characterized by tremor, rigidity, bradykinesia and postural instability, are two subtypes of progressive heterogeneous neurodegenerative diseases with Parkinsonism as a representative feature [3]. And neuroimaging holds great promise in accurate diagnosing and staging of early, new onset and prodromal PD [4]. Imaging biomarkers with multimodal quantifications could visualize structural and functional brain changes that might help revealing the underlying pathophysiological abnormalities in PD [5]. For instance, hybrid PET/MRI was used for exploring the coupling between resting-state fMRI and dopamine release quantified with PET molecular tracer such as

[^{11}-C]raclopride for PD patients with motor complications, and also for evaluation of neuroprotective treatment efficacy [6].

Multiple brain circuits including limbic and mesolimbic pathways had demonstrated widespread functional and metabolic abnormalities in the orbitofrontal, anterior cingulate, amygdala, thalamus and ventral striatum (VST) that might account for the neuropsychiatric disorders such as depression, anxiety and apathy in PD [7]. Perfusion network analysis identified blood flow differences in the medial temporal lobe between PD and Alzheimer's disease (AD) patients, with both showing hypoperfusion in the posterior cingulate cortex (PCC), precuneus and visual cortex compared to controls [8]. Nigrosome-1 imaging for quantification of loss of nigrosome-1 (N1) dopaminergic neurons in the N1 territory in SN has made progress with high resolution MRI and more validation studies [9]. And N1-sign was observed either unilaterally or bilaterally in majorities of Parkinsonism and related disorders using susceptibility weighted imaging (SWI) with high spatial resolution [10]. Finally, significant changes of susceptibility values of lower than 70 pars per billion (ppb) in idiopathic PD patients compared to healthy controls (HC) were observed in SN area using SWI together with the histogram analysis [11].

Striatal dopamine transporters (DAT) in the caudate/putamen regions and vesicular monoamine transporter type 2 (VMAT2) binding densities with PET/SPECT molecular tracers such as Ioflupane[^{123}I] and [^{18}F]AV-133 had been evaluated for dopamine synthesis, storage and pathway analyses [12, 13]. Several studies had reported concentration differences of DAT and VMAT2 in PD compared to controls. For 6 regions of interest (ROIs) in the caudate and putamen, lower DAT availability was observed; and left anterior putamen DAT availability was correlated to the anxiety and depression symptoms in patients [14]. PD patients with impulse control disorder (ICD) had significantly lower DAT density in the VST than PD without ICD, and DAT was associated with ICD severity that might account for dysfunction of some related cortico-subcortical networks [15]. In the nigrostriatal and basal ganglia systems, DAT was severally reduced in the dorsal putamen (DPU), then in the ventral tegmental area (VTA) and with a less degree in the SN and VST [16]. Also a derangement of nigrostriatal pathway between the SN and DPU dopamine network connectivity was found additionally. And the striatal dopamine denervation, such as reduced kinetic parameter K(i) in the putamen, might contribute to some frontostriatal cognitive impairment in moderate stage of PD [17]. Furthermore, VMAT2 densities in PCC, left caudate, anterior putamen and VST were associated with cerebrospinal fluid (CSF) Aβ1–42 level, and VMAT2 in the SN/left VST were related to CSF total/phosphorylated tau levels respectively [18].

In addition to the multiparametric MRI results of PD and several subgroups in Chapter 1, the purpose of this section is to reveal the PET molecular imaging abnormalities in these patients, including the DAT and striatal binding ratio (SBR) data, as well as the cortico-subcortical VMAT2 pathway quantifications with ROI analysis.

1.2. Methods and Data

MRI/PET Imaging data used in the preparation of this article were obtained from the ADNI database (http://ida.loni.usc.edu). The primary goal of ADNI has been to test whether serial MRI, positron emission tomography (PET), other biological markers, and clinical and neuropsychological assessment can be combined to measure the progression of mild cognitive impairment (MCI) and early Alzheimer's disease (AD). ADNI is the result of efforts of many co-investigators from a broad range of academic institutions and private corporations, and subjects have been recruited from over 50 sites across the United States and Canada. For up-to- date information, see www.adni-info.org.

Preprocessed PET molecular imaging data of the most recent date were downloaded from the Parkinson's Progression Markers Initiative (PPMI) program as one of the ADNI centers. PET tracer, 9-[18F]fluoropropyl-(+)-dihydrotetrabenazine ([^{18}F]AV-133), was used to target VMAT2 distribution in the central nervous system. A total of 34 regions were evaluated including cerebellum, bilateral sub-cortical and cortical regions such as caudate, orbitofrontal and occipital cortices. AV-133 measuring

SBR was post-analyzed for comparisons between sub-groups of PD such as PD from general cohort (GPD, slightly more severe than PD) and prodromal (PM) patients in bilateral caudate, anterior and posterior putamen portions. DAT data were evaluated in two striatal regions including bilateral caudate and putamen.

1.3. Results

Significantly lower striatal binding ratio (SBR) in the PD compared to normal controls (NC) in bilateral caudate (CAUD, $P < 0.006$), anterior putamen (PUTANT, $P < 0.0002$), and posterior putamen (PUTPOST, $P < 0.000001$) were identified (Table1). Comparing PD patients to controls, the percentage reduction of dopamine SBR was in the range of -[33-71]% with mean of -53% reduction in PD. Furthermore, lower dopamine transporter (DAT) levels in both PD and GPD compared to NC were found in the striatum regions such as bilateral caudate and putamen ($P < 0.0001$) (Table 2). Lower DAT levels in the GPD compared to PD were also present in these four ROIs, with slightly less significance level ($P < 0.007$) (Table 2). In comparison to controls, the average percentage reduction of DAT level in the caudate and putamen region was -41% and -62% respectively for PD patients, together with -46% and -69% for GPD patients.

Statistical comparisons between groups of VMAT2 densities are listed in Table 3. Significantly lower VMAT2 levels in prodromal (PM) patients compared to healthy controls (HC) were found in multiple brain regions including bilateral mesial temporal cortex, left caudate, parietal and occipital cortices with $P < 0.05$. Similarly lower VMAT2 levels in bilateral mesial temporal cortex, orbitofrontal cortex including rectus were observed in the PD compared to NC (generally unaffected) ($P < 0.02$). Multiple brain regions also presented significantly lower VMAT2 levels comparing PM group to NC, such as bilateral mesial temporal cortex, caudate, orbitofrontal cortex, left frontal and occipital cortices ($P < 0.04$). Additionally PM patients had lower VMAT2 levels in regions of bilateral occipital, left temporal and caudate compared to PD group, as well as lower VMAT2 levels in bilateral occipital and left mesial temporal cortex compared to GPD group (both P < 0.05).

Table 1. AV-133 measuring striatal binding ratio (SBR) change in PD compared to NC. Percentage change (%) = (PD-NC)/NC*100%

ROI	NC	PD	P-value	Percentage Change (%)
RCAUD	2.164 ± 0.098	1.398 ± 0.104	0.005526	-35
RPUTANT	2.636 ± 0.146	1.250 ± 0.130	0.000154	-53
RPUTPOST	2.388 ± 0.117	0.713 ± 0.101	< 0.000001	-70
LCAUD	2.086 ± 0.131	1.390 ± 0.087	0.003145	-33
LPUTANT	2.580 ± 0.171	1.226 ± 0.093	0.000002	-52
LPUTPOST	2.394 ± 0.144	0.693 ± 0.083	< 0.000001	-71

* Significantly lower striatal binding ratio (SBR) in the PD compared to NC were found in bilateral left (L) and right (R) caudate (CAUD, P < 0.006), anterior putamen (PUTANT, P < 0.0002), and posterior putamen (PUTPOST, P < 0.000001). The percentage reduction was in the range of -[33-71] % with mean of -53% reduction of SBR in PD patients compared to NC.

Table 2. Dopamine transporter (DAT) level differences in three groups including PD, GPD and NC in bilateral caudate and putamen

ROI	Mean ± Std			Comparison		
	1-NC	2-PD	3-GPD	P (1,2)	P (1,3)	P (2,3)
CAUDATE_R	2.949 ± 0.043	1.758 ± 0.032	1.579 ± 0.043	<0.0001	<0.0001	0.0015
CAUDATE_L	2.985 ± 0.044	1.753 ± 0.032	1.601 ± 0.041	<0.0001	<0.0001	0.0063
PUTAMEN_R	2.132 ± 0.040	0.827 ± 0.026	0.662 ± 0.026	<0.0001	<0.0001	0.0001
PUTAMEN_L	2.134 ± 0.039	0.810 ± 0.026	0.681 ± 0.023	<0.0001	<0.0001	0.0025

* Significantly lower dopamine transporter (DAT) levels in PD and GPD compared to NC were observed in the striatum regions such as bilateral caudate and putamen (all P < 0.0001). Lower DAT levels in the GPD compared to PD were also present in these four ROIs (P < 0.007). P(1,2) indicates P-value comparing PD (group 2) to NC (group 1), and P(1,3) for comparing GPD (group 3) to NC, P(2,3) for comparison between GPD and PD. The average percentage reduction of DAT level in the caudate and putamen region was -41% and -62% respectively for PD patients, -46% and -69% for GPD patients compared to controls.

The range of VMAT2 reduction in PD/GPD/PM was -[1-11.6] % with mean of -6.1 ± 0.4%, and lowest relative reduction of -11.6% was found in the left caudate comparing prodromal group to healthy controls.

Table 3. VMAT2 density comparison in pairs of five groups; with indexes coded as: 1-HC; 2- normal controls (NC) from general cohort unaffected individuals (GENUN); 3-Prodromal (PM); 4-PD; 5-GPD

ROI	Group 1	Group 2	Comparison	P-value
mean whole cerebellum	1.087 ± 0.005	1.076 ± 0.003	P(1,5)	0.0440
mesial temporal cortex r	1.306 ± 0.039	1.209 ± 0.028	P(1,3)	0.0485
mesial temporal cortex l	1.277 ± 0.033	1.189 ± 0.024	P(1,3)	0.0359
caudate l	1.436 ± 0.053	1.269 ± 0.046	P(1,3)	0.0228
occipital cortex l	1.377 ± 0.042	1.276 ± 0.023	P(1,3)	0.0399
parietal cortex l	1.327 ± 0.038	1.235 ± 0.024	P(1,3)	0.0420
lateral temporal cortex l	1.287 ± 0.037	1.194 ± 0.023	P(1,3)	0.0352
temporal cortex l	1.284 ± 0.035	1.194 ± 0.022	P(1,3)	0.0322
mean whole cerebellum	1.087 ± 0.005	1.072 ± 0.003	P(1,3)	0.0168
mesial temporal cortex r	1.302 ± 0.019	1.246 ± 0.015	P(2,4)	0.0243
mesial temporal cortex l	1.297 ± 0.018	1.239 ± 0.015	P(2,4)	0.0187
subcortical white matter	2.222 ± 0.042	2.093 ± 0.036	P(2,4)	0.0243
cerebellar white matter	2.287 ± 0.037	2.160 ± 0.034	P(2,4)	0.0180
rectus l	1.358 ± 0.018	1.277 ± 0.020	P(2,4)	0.0059
orbitofrontal cortex l	1.339 ± 0.017	1.272 ± 0.017	P(2,4)	0.0120
cerebellar cortex r	0.993 ± 0.004	1.009 ± 0.006	P(2,3)	0.0336
cerebellar cortex l	1.007 ± 0.004	0.991 ± 0.006	P(2,3)	0.0258
mesial temporal cortex r	1.302 ± 0.019	1.209 ± 0.028	P(2,3)	0.0071
mesial temporal cortex l	1.297 ± 0.018	1.189 ± 0.024	P(2,3)	0.0007
subcortical white matter	2.222 ± 0.042	2.004 ± 0.059	P(2,3)	0.0034
cerebellar white matter	2.287 ± 0.037	2.068 ± 0.059	P(2,3)	0.0020
rectus l	1.358 ± 0.018	1.262 ± 0.034	P(2,3)	0.0098
caudate r	1.499 ± 0.031	1.362 ± 0.044	P(2,3)	0.0129
caudate l	1.416 ± 0.030	1.269 ± 0.046	P(2,3)	0.0083
occipital cortex l	1.342 ± 0.019	1.276 ± 0.023	P(2,3)	0.0350
lateral temporal cortex l	1.260 ± 0.017	1.194 ± 0.023	P(2,3)	0.0202
orbitofrontal cortex r	1.323 ± 0.018	1.242 ± 0.034	P(2,3)	0.0273
orbitofrontal cortex l	1.339 ± 0.017	1.239 ± 0.034	P(2,3)	0.0064
frontal cortex l	1.384 ± 0.022	1.298 ± 0.030	P(2,3)	0.0225
temporal cortex l	1.269 ± 0.016	1.194 ± 0.022	P(2,3)	0.0078
caudate l	1.391 ± 0.025	1.269 ± 0.046	P(4,3)	0.0149
occipital cortex r	1.341 ± 0.018	1.275 ± 0.023	P(4,3)	0.0375
occipital cortex l	1.360 ± 0.018	1.276 ± 0.023	P(4,3)	0.0111
parietal cortex l	1.310 ± 0.022	1.235 ± 0.024	P(4,3)	0.0469
lateral temporal cortex l	1.261 ± 0.016	1.194 ± 0.023	P(4,3)	0.0251

Table 3. (Continued)

ROI	Group 1	Group 2	Comparison	P-value
temporal cortex l	1.256 ± 0.016	1.194 ± 0.022	P(4,3)	0.0331
mesial temporal cortex l	1.263 ± 0.021	1.189 ± 0.024	P(5,3)	0.0279
occipital cortex r	1.343 ± 0.022	1.275 ± 0.023	P(5,3)	0.0451
occipital cortex l	1.358 ± 0.027	1.276 ± 0.023	P(5,3)	0.0372

Significant results included lower VMAT2 levels in prodromal (PM, group 3) patients compared to HC (group 1) were found in multiple brain regions including bilateral mesial temporal cortex, left caudate, parietal and occipital cortices, as P(1,3) < 0.05 in the last two columns. Lower VMAT2 in bilateral mesial temporal cortex, orbitofrontal cortex including rectus were observed in PD (group 4) compared to NC (generally unaffected) (group 2) (P(2,4) < 0.02). Multiple brain regions also presented significantly lower VMAT2 levels comparing PM group to NC (generally unaffected), such as bilateral mesial temporal cortex, caudate, orbitofrontal cortex, left frontal and occipital cortices (P(2,3) < 0.04). Additionally PM patients had lower VMAT2 levels in regions of bilateral occipital, left temporal and caudate compared to PD group (P(4,3) < 0.05). And finally, PM group also had lower VMAT2 levels in bilateral occipital and left mesial temporal cortex compared to GPD (group 5) (P(3,5) < 0.05).

*l = left; r = right; 1-HC; 2-normal controls (NC) from general cohort unaffected individuals (GENUN); 3-Prodromal (PM); 4-PD; 5-GPD. Lower VMAT2 densities were present in Group 2 compared to Group 1 in almost all regions, with the only exception of right cerebellar cortex. The percentage reduction was in the range of -[1-11.6] % with mean of -6.1 ± 0.4% reduction of VMAT2 densities in group 2 compared to group 1. Lowest relative reduction of -11.6% was found in the left caudate comparing prodromal group to healthy controls.

Taken together, expected lower SBR and DAT levels in PD compared to NC were found in the striatal caudate and putamen regions. Generally, less VMAT2 densities in PD/GPD compared to NC were found in regions of bilateral mesial temporal cortex, caudate, orbitofrontal cortex, left frontal and occipital cortices; however with a lower level in PM compared to other groups were observed additionally. The PET molecular imaging results were in line with the pervious MRI results including structural morphology, fMRI resting state interhemispheric coordination, functional connectivity maps using dual regression and microstructural DTI results. Specifically, the PET molecular imaging results, showing reduced dopamine transporter and binding potential levels in striatum together with less cortical (spare of parietal lobe) and caudate dopamine storage and pathway deficits, were in line with the MRI imaging results including swallow tail sign signature (dopaminergic neuron reductions in nigrosome-1 territory) in the substantia nigra with less microstructural connectivity or conductivity, gray matter atrophy and lower interhemispheric coordination/ functional connectivity in the inferior/middle temporal, occipital and medial-orbito frontal cortices as well.

1.4. Discussion and Treatment of PD

Our consistent PET/MRI results, showing dopamine deficits (~50% SBR and DAT reduction) in the SN, as well as cortical orbito-frontal, temporal and occipital dysfunction in PD/GPD/PM patients compared to controls, reflected multi-domain brain functional abnormalities such as motor, learning and memory problems and possible depression in PD patients. The motor disturbance in PD is thought to be related to the dopamine deficiency [19]. The estimated SN dopamine neurons damage could reach 60%-80% over a period of ~5 to 15 years before symptoms emerge [20]. Although replacing or boosting existing dopamine levels could be used to monitor disease progression, the therapeutic benefits might be limited. Pharmacotherapy such as levodopa (L-DOPA) including new formulations and dopamine agonists, deep brain stimulation (DBS) and physiotherapy are commonly used for treating the motor symptoms of PD [21]. Progressive disability in PD corresponds only to symptomatic therapy, and chronic pharmacotherapy (especially with dopamine receptor agonists) might cause impulse compulsive disorder (ICD) in patients [22, 23]. Also dopaminergic treatment could trigger nonmotor behavior symptom including affective disorders, as the basal ganglia has functionally connected with a few brain regions such as the orbitofrontal cortex and mesolimbic circuit [24].

MRI imaging evaluation of the L-DOPA treatment found that the connectivity between cerebellar brain regions and subcortical areas of the motor system such as the thalamus/putamen increased and correlated with improved clinical symptoms such as the Unified Parkinson's Disease Rating Scale (UPDRS) motor score [25]. Disruption of functional connectivity of MRI (fcMRI) between cortical and subcortical structures during virtual reality paradigm for freezing of gait evaluation was found in

PD patients [26]. Patients in the dopamine depletion OFF state had lower apraxia scores than controls, together with lower fcMRI between the supramarginal gyrus and the primary motor cortex, basal ganglia, and frontal areas than ON state [27]. Also greater network-level integration (i.e., global efficiency) in PD was found in the dopaminergic OFF state than ON state based on fcMRI data, and was inversely related to motor symptom severity for possible compensation. The increased global efficiency had been further connected with cognitive and brain reserve in the depletion OFF state [28].

For the DBS treatment evaluation, DBS in the subthalamic nucleus (STN) using the direct MRI-based targeting (dTM) for reducing motor fluctuation and overcoming side effects of medication, had resulted in significant improvement in majorities of PD patients [29]. For instance, the UPDRS scores were better, and dyskinesias as well as fluctuations were both reduced at twelve months after dTM STN DBS treatment. dTM STN In addition, DBS were validated as a powerful tool for treating both motor and coordination dysfunction with better clinical outcome such as improved connectivity between STN and motor/premotor areas [30-32]. And it had also been found that transcranial magnetic stimulation (TMS) for treating depression symptom in PD resulted in balanced functional connectivity of dorsolateral prefrontal cortex while fluoxetine resulted in enhanced medial prefrontal fcMRI [33].

2. PET/MRI Application in Brain Science and Neurological Diseases

2.1. PET/MRI in Brain Science

PET/MRI can also be utilized to investigate simultaneous neuroscience processes in brain and reveal the differences affected with multiple physiological and neuropathological factors [34-37]. For instance, in the aging brain, women had more gray matter densities measured with MRI structural voxel-based morphometry (VBM) algorithm in multiple brain regions than men. These regions included medial orbito-frontal and prefrontal cortices, middle temporal cortex such as hippocampus and fusiform, middle occipital region, superior and inferior parietal clusters, supramarginal gyrus, primary and associated somatosensory cortices, motor and supplementary motor clusters (Figure 1A).

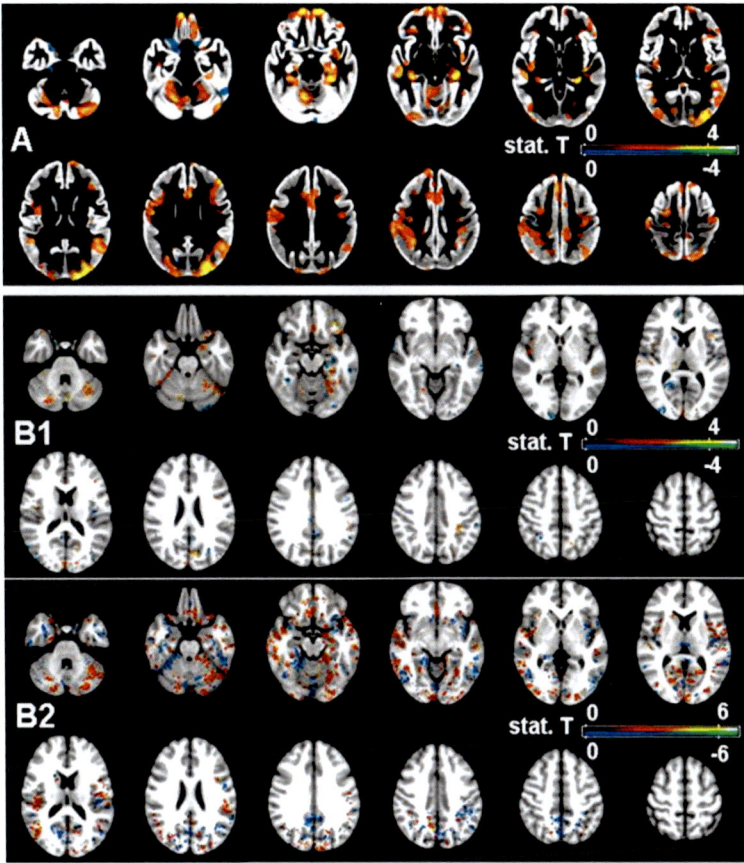

Figure 1. PET/MRI integration results: gender differences in adults showing less gray matter density (A) and more neuropathological amyloid burden correlation in men (B2) compared to women (B1). Color indicates significant gray matter density difference of corrected $P < 0.05$ (statistical T value ≥ 2) in A, and significant correlation between MRI gray matter density with VBM and PET PiB amyloid deposition with corrected $P < 0.05$ in B1 & B2.

In line with these findings, women also had less neuropathological correspondence with amyloid deposition imaged with PET PiB tracer in brain, with the correlation map between gray matter density and amyloid deposition shown in Figure 1 B1 for women and Figure 1 B2 for men respectively. Specifically, men had more regional amyloid accumulation correlations with gray matter density in the temporal cortex including parahippocampus and middle temporal lobe, lingual and calcarine cortex, insular, rolandic operculum, supramarginal gyrus, medial orbito-frontal cortex and rectus, and cerebellum than women (mainly positive correlation in hot color with corrected $P < 0.05$ in Figure 1B). Some brain regions including the precuneus, small clusters in the visual and temporal cortices also demonstrated more negative association between gray matter density and amyloid accumulation in men than women (Figure 1B, cold color with corrected $P < 0.05$).

In summary, our representative examples demonstrated multiparametric quantifications with the integrated PET/MRI modalities for the neurodegenerative disease and biological factor investigation in brain science. Our results were consistent with reported findings with either single modality or combined modalities [38-40], and could help interpret the underlying co-existing pathophysiological processes in both brain and whole-body biological systems.

2.2. PET/MRI in Neurological Diseases

Simultaneous PET/MRI had been utilized to study complex brain functions for monitoring multiple biological signals at various conditions such as task processing or in response to pharmacological interventions with high spatiotemporal resolution [41]. In neurodegenerative diseases, PET/MRI might provide better diagnosis with multiple advanced imaging quantifications and intrinsic co-registration of two imaging modalities, including Parkinson's disease (PD) and Alzheimer's disease (AD) [42]. Simultaneous cerebral blood flow and metabolism changes in superficial temporal artery-middle cerebral artery (STA-MCA) bypass surgery could be demonstrated using both MRI arterial spin labeling (ASL) and PET FDG-glucose quantifications [43]. Similarly, in frontotemporal dementia (FTD), hypoperfusion and hypometabolism measured with PET/MRI were consistent, with different degrees involved due to distinct neurophysiology of the two metrics [44]. Neuroinflammation measured with PET [^{11}C]-PBR28 tracer correlated well with MRI brain atrophy and showed high signal-to-background ratio in Huntington's disease [45]. Neuropathological tau burden correlated with gray matter atrophy, and was associated with cognitive performance test in AD [46, 47]. Other neurologic applications had been reported with combined PET and MRI molecular, structural and functional imaging features, such as in the areas of therapeutic assessments and early disease prevention [48]. More accurate quantification, synchronous pathophysiology investigation and consistent cross-validation could be achieved with advanced PET/MRI imaging techniques, including fast reconstruction with improved attenuation correction at higher spatiotemporal resolutions for better integration and correlation with other biomarkers including multiomics and general clinical applications in various diseases [49-54].

REFERENCES

[1] Shih MC, Hoexter MQ, Andrade LA, Bressan RA. Parkinson's disease and dopamine transporter neuroimaging: a critical review. *Sao Paulo Med J.* 2006 May 4;124(3):168-75. doi: 10.1590/s1516-31802006000300014. PMID: 17119698.

[2] Weingarten CP, Sundman MH, Hickey P, Chen NK. Neuroimaging of Parkinson's disease: Expanding views. *Neurosci Biobehav Rev.* 2015 Dec;59:16-52. doi: 10.1016/j.neubiorev.2015.09.007. Epub 2015 Sep 26. PMID: 26409344; PMCID: PMC4763948.

[3] Saeed U, Lang AE, Masellis M. Neuroimaging Advances in Parkinson's Disease and Atypical Parkinsonian Syndromes. *Front Neurol.* 2020 Oct 15;11:572976. doi: 10.3389/fneur.2020.572976. PMID: 33178113; PMCID: PMC7593544.

[4] Heim B, Krismer F, De Marzi R, Seppi K. Magnetic resonance imaging for the diagnosis of Parkinson's disease. *J Neural Transm (Vienna).* 2017 Aug;124(8):915-964. doi: 10.1007/s00702-017-1717-8. Epub 2017 Apr 4. PMID: 28378231; PMCID: PMC5514207.

[5] Saeed U, Compagnone J, Aviv RI, Strafella AP, Black SE, Lang AE, Masellis M. Imaging biomarkers in Parkinson's disease and Parkinsonian syndromes: current and emerging concepts. *Transl Neurodegener.* 2017 Mar 28;6:8. doi: 10.1186/s40035-017-0076-6. PMID: 28360997; PMCID: PMC5370489.

[6] Tondo G, Esposito M, Dervenoulas G, Wilson H, Politis M, Pagano G. Hybrid PET-MRI Applications in Movement Disorders. *Int Rev Neurobiol.* 2019;144:211-257. doi: 10.1016/bs.irn.2018.10.003. Epub 2018 Nov 8. PMID: 30638455.

[7] Thobois S, Prange S, Sgambato-Faure V, Tremblay L, Broussolle E. Imaging the Etiology of Apathy, Anxiety, and Depression in Parkinson's Disease: Implication for Treatment. *Curr Neurol Neurosci Rep.* 2017 Aug 18;17(10):76. doi: 10.1007/s11910-017-0788-0. PMID: 28822071.

[8] Le Heron CJ, Wright SL, Melzer TR, Myall DJ, MacAskill MR, Livingston L, Keenan RJ, Watts R, Dalrymple-Alford JC, Anderson TJ. Comparing cerebral perfusion in Alzheimer's disease and Parkinson's disease dementia: an ASL-MRI study. *J Cereb Blood Flow Metab.* 2014 Jun;34(6):964-70. doi: 10.1038/jcbfm.2014.40. Epub 2014 Mar 12. PMID: 24619276; PMCID: PMC4050238.

[9] Kim EY, Sung YH, Lee J. Nigrosome 1 imaging: technical considerations and clinical applications. *Br J Radiol.* 2019 Sep;92 (1101): 20180842. doi: 10.1259/bjr.20180842. Epub 2019 Jun 5. PMID: 31067082; PMCID: PMC6732928.

[10] Cheng Z, He N, Huang P, Li Y, Tang R, Sethi SK, Ghassaban K, Yerramsetty KK, Palutla VK, Chen S, Yan F, Haacke EM. Imaging the Nigrosome 1 in the substantia nigra using susceptibility weighted imaging and quantitative susceptibility mapping: An application to Parkinson's disease. *Neuroimage Clin.* 2020;25:102103. doi:

10.1016/j.nicl.2019.102103. Epub 2019 Nov 20. PMID: 31869769; PMCID: PMC6933220.

[11] Kim EY, Sung YH, Shin HG, Noh Y, Nam Y, Lee J. Diagnosis of Early-Stage Idiopathic Parkinson's Disease Using High-Resolution Quantitative Susceptibility Mapping Combined with Histogram Analysis in the Substantia Nigra at 3 T. *J Clin Neurol.* 2018 Jan;14(1):90-97. doi: 10.3988/jcn.2018.14.1.90. PMID: 29629545; PMCID: PMC5765262.

[12] Felicio AC, Shih MC, Godeiro-Junior C, Andrade LA, Bressan RA, Ferraz HB. Molecular imaging studies in Parkinson disease: reducing diagnostic uncertainty. *Neurologist.* 2009 Jan;15(1):6-16. doi: 10.1097/NRL.0b013e318183fdd8. PMID: 19131852.

[13] Arena JE, Stoessl AJ. Optimizing diagnosis in Parkinson's disease: Radionuclide imaging. *Parkinsonism Relat Disord.* 2016 Jan;22 Suppl 1:S47-51. doi: 10.1016/j.parkreldis.2015.09.029. Epub 2015 Sep 15. PMID: 26439947.

[14] Weintraub D, Newberg AB, Cary MS, Siderowf AD, Moberg PJ, Kleiner-Fisman G, Duda JE, Stern MB, Mozley D, Katz IR. Striatal dopamine transporter imaging correlates with anxiety and depression symptoms in Parkinson's disease. J Nucl Med. 2005 Feb;46(2):227-32. PMID: 15695780.

[15] Navalpotro-Gomez I, Dacosta-Aguayo R, Molinet-Dronda F, Martin-Bastida A, Botas-Peñin A, Jimenez-Urbieta H, Delgado-Alvarado M, Gago B, Quiroga-Varela A, Rodriguez-Oroz MC. Nigrostriatal dopamine transporter availability, and its metabolic and clinical correlates in Parkinson's disease patients with impulse control disorders. *Eur J Nucl Med Mol Imaging.* 2019 Sep; 46(10): 2065-2076. doi: 10.1007/s00259-019-04396-3. Epub 2019 Jul 4. PMID: 31273436.

[16] Caminiti SP, Presotto L, Baroncini D, Garibotto V, Moresco RM, Gianolli L, Volonté MA, Antonini A, Perani D. Axonal damage and loss of connectivity in nigrostriatal and mesolimbic dopamine pathways in early Parkinson's disease. *Neuroimage Clin.* 2017 Mar

27;14:734-740. doi: 10.1016/j.nicl.2017.03.011. PMID: 28409113; PMCID: PMC5379906.

[17] Cropley VL, Fujita M, Bara-Jimenez W, Brown AK, Zhang XY, Sangare J, Herscovitch P, Pike VW, Hallett M, Nathan PJ, Innis RB. Pre- and post-synaptic dopamine imaging and its relation with frontostriatal cognitive function in Parkinson disease: PET studies with [11C]NNC 112 and [18F]FDOPA. *Psychiatry Res.* 2008 Jul 15;163(2):171-82. doi: 10.1016/j.pscychresns. 2007.11.003. Epub 2008 May 27. PMID: 18504119.

[18] Gao R, Zhang G, Chen X, Yang A, Smith G, Wong DF, Zhou Y. CSF Biomarkers and Its Associations with 18F-AV133 Cerebral VMAT2 Binding in Parkinson's Disease-A Preliminary Report. *PLoS One.* 2016 Oct 20;11(10):e0164762. doi: 10.1371/journal. pone.0164762. PMID: 27764160; PMCID: PMC5072678.

[19] Delenclos M, Jones DR, McLean PJ, Uitti RJ. Biomarkers in Parkinson's disease: Advances and strategies. *Parkinsonism Relat Disord.* 2016 Jan;22 Suppl 1(Suppl 1):S106-10. doi: 10.1016/j. parkreldis.2015.09.048. Epub 2015 Sep 30. PMID: 26439946; PMCID: PMC5120398.

[20] Miller DB, O'Callaghan JP. Biomarkers of Parkinson's disease: present and future. *Metabolism.* 2015 Mar;64(3 Suppl 1):S40-6. doi: 10.1016/j.metabol.2014.10.030. Epub 2014 Oct 31. PMID: 25510818; PMCID: PMC4721253.

[21] Oertel W, Schulz JB. Current and experimental treatments of Parkinson disease: A guide for neuroscientists. *J Neurochem.* 2016 Oct;139 Suppl 1:325-337. doi: 10.1111/jnc.13750. Epub 2016 Aug 30. PMID: 27577098.

[22] Cova I, Priori A. Diagnostic biomarkers for Parkinson's disease at a glance: where are we? *J Neural Transm (Vienna).* 2018 Oct;125(10): 1417-1432. doi: 10.1007/s00702-018-1910-4. Epub 2018 Aug 25. PMID: 30145631; PMCID: PMC6132920.

[23] Roussakis AA, Lao-Kaim NP, Piccini P. Brain Imaging and Impulse Control Disorders in Parkinson's Disease. *Curr Neurol Neurosci*

Rep. 2019 Aug 8;19(9):67. doi: 10.1007/s11910-019-0980-5. PMID: 31396719; PMCID: PMC6689903.

[24] minian KS, Strafella AP. Affective disorders in Parkinson's disease. *Curr Opin Neurol.* 2013 Aug;26(4):339-44. doi: 10.1097/WCO. 0b013e328363304c. PMID: 23757262; PMCID: PMC4452223.

[25] Mueller K, Jech R, Ballarini T, Holiga Š, Růžička F, Piecha FA, Möller HE, Vymazal J, Růžička E, Schroeter ML. Modulatory Effects of Levodopa on Cerebellar Connectivity in Parkinson's Disease. *Cerebellum.* 2019 Apr;18(2):212-224. doi: 10.1007/s12311-018-0981-y. PMID: 30298443; PMCID: PMC6443641.

[26] Bluett B, Bayram E, Litvan I. The virtual reality of Parkinson's disease freezing of gait: A systematic review. *Parkinsonism Relat Disord.* 2019 Apr;61:26-33. doi: 10.1016/j.parkreldis.2018.11.013. Epub 2018 Nov 15. PMID: 30470656; PMCID: PMC6773254.

[27] Matt E, Fischmeister FPS, Foki T, Beisteiner R. Dopaminergic modulation of the praxis network in Parkinson's disease. *Neuroimage Clin.* 2019;24:101988. doi: 10.1016/j.nicl.2019.101988. Epub 2019 Aug 18. PMID: 31479896; PMCID: PMC6726913.

[28] Shine JM, Bell PT, Matar E, Poldrack RA, Lewis SJG, Halliday GM, O'Callaghan C. Dopamine depletion alters macroscopic network dynamics in Parkinson's disease. *Brain.* 2019 Apr 1;142(4):1024-1034. doi: 10.1093/brain/awz034. PMID: 30887035; PMCID: PMC6904322.

[29] Lahtinen MJ, Haapaniemi TH, Kauppinen MT, Salokorpi N, Heikkinen ER, Katisko JP. A comparison of indirect and direct targeted STN DBS in the treatment of Parkinson's disease-surgical method and clinical outcome over 15-year timespan. *Acta Neurochir (Wien).* 2020 May;162(5):1067-1076. doi: 10.1007/s00701-020-04269-x. Epub 2020 Feb 26. PMID: 32103343; PMCID: PMC7156355.

[30] Horn A, Reich M, Vorwerk J, Li N, Wenzel G, Fang Q, Schmitz-Hübsch T, Nickl R, Kupsch A, Volkmann J, Kühn AA, Fox MD. Connectivity Predicts deep brain stimulation outcome in Parkinson

disease. *Ann Neurol.* 2017 Jul;82(1):67-78. doi: 10.1002/ana.24974. PMID: 28586141; PMCID: PMC5880678.

[31] Schulz JB, Hausmann L, Hardy J. 199 years of Parkinson disease - what have we learned and what is the path to the future? *J Neurochem.* 2016 Oct;139 Suppl 1:3-7. doi: 10.1111/jnc.13733. Epub 2016 Aug 31. PMID: 27581372.

[32] Albaugh DL, Shih YY. Neural circuit modulation during deep brain stimulation at the subthalamic nucleus for Parkinson's disease: what have we learned from neuroimaging studies? *Brain Connect.* 2014 Feb;4(1):1-14. doi: 10.1089/brain.2013.0193. Epub 2013 Dec 18. PMID: 24147633; PMCID: PMC5349222.

[33] Cardoso EF, Fregni F, Martins Maia F, Boggio PS, Luis Myczkowski M, Coracini K, Lopes Vieira A, Melo LM, Sato JR, Antonio Marcolin M, Rigonatti SP, Cruz AC Jr, Reis Barbosa E, Amaro E Jr. rTMS treatment for depression in Parkinson's disease increases BOLD responses in the left prefrontal cortex. *Int J Neuropsychopharmacol.* 2008 Mar;11(2):173-83. doi: 10.1017/ S1461145707007961. *Epub 2007 Aug* 21. PMID: 17708780.

[34] Zhou Y. *Functional Neuroimaging with Multiple Modalities: Principle, Device and Applicaitons.* Nova Science Publishers. 2016.

[35] Fox PT, Raichle ME, Mintun MA, Dence C. Nonoxidative glucose consumption during focal physiologic neural activity. *Science.* 1988;241(4864):462-464.

[36] Apostolova LG, Thompson PM. Brain mapping as a tool to study neurodegeneration. *Neurotherapeutics.* 2007 Jul;4(3):387-400.

[37] Zhou Y, Qiu L, Sterpka A, Wang H, Chu F, Chen X. Comparative Phosphoproteomic Profiling of Type III Adenylyl Cyclase Knockout and Control, Male, and Female Mice. *Front Cell Neurosci.* 2019 Feb 13;13:34. doi: 10.3389/fncel.2019.00034. PMID: 30814930; PMCID: PMC6381875.

[38] Xin J, Zhang Y, Tang Y, Yang Y. Brain Differences Between Men and Women: Evidence From Deep Learning. *Front Neurosci.* 2019 Mar 8;13:185.

[39] Curiati PK, Tamashiro JH, Squarzoni P, Duran FL, Santos LC, Wajngarten M, Leite CC, Vallada H, Menezes PR, Scazufca M, Busatto GF, Alves TC. Brain structural variability due to aging and gender in cognitively healthy Elders: results from the Sao Paulo Ageing and Health study. *AJNR Am J Neuroradiol.* 2009 Nov;30(10):1850-6.

[40] Lotze M, Domin M, Gerlach FH, Gaser C, Lueders E, Schmidt CO, Neumann N. Novel findings from 2,838 Adult Brains on Sex Differences in Gray Matter Brain Volume. *Sci Rep.* 2019 Feb 8;9(1):1671.

[41] Werner P, Barthel H, Drzezga A, Sabri O. Current status and future role of brain PET/MRI in clinical and research settings. *Eur J Nucl Med Mol Imaging.* 2015 Mar;42(3):512-26. doi: 10.1007/s00259-014-2970-9. Epub 2015 Jan 9. PMID: 25573629.

[42] Hope TA, Fayad ZA, Fowler KJ, Holley D, Iagaru A, McMillan AB, Veit-Haiback P, Witte RJ, Zaharchuk G, Catana C. Summary of the First ISMRM-SNMMI Workshop on PET/MRI: Applications and Limitations. *J Nucl Med.* 2019 Oct;60(10):1340-1346. doi: 10.2967/jnumed.119.227231. Epub 2019 May 23. PMID: 31123099; PMCID: PMC6785790.

[43] Cui B, Zhang T, Ma Y, Chen Z, Ma J, Ma L, Jiao L, Zhou Y, Shan B, Lu J. Simultaneous PET-MRI imaging of cerebral blood flow and glucose metabolism in the symptomatic unilateral internal carotid artery/middle cerebral artery steno-occlusive disease. *Eur J Nucl Med Mol Imaging.* 2020 Jul;47(7):1668-1677. doi: 10.1007/s00259-019-04551-w. Epub 2019 Nov 6. PMID: 31691843; PMCID: PMC7248051.

[44] Anazodo UC, Finger E, Kwan BYM, Pavlosky W, Warrington JC, Günther M, Prato FS, Thiessen JD, St Lawrence KS. Using simultaneous PET/MRI to compare the accuracy of diagnosing frontotemporal dementia by arterial spin labelling MRI and FDG-PET. *Neuroimage Clin.* 2017 Oct 31;17:405-414. doi: 10.1016/j.nicl.2017.10.033. PMID: 29159053; PMCID: PMC5683801.

[45] Lois C, González I, Izquierdo-García D, Zürcher NR, Wilkens P, Loggia ML, Hooker JM, Rosas HD. Neuroinflammation in Huntington's Disease: New Insights with 11C-PBR28 PET/MRI. *ACS Chem Neurosci.* 2018 Nov 21;9(11):2563-2571. doi: 10.1021/acschemneuro. 8b00072. Epub 2018 May 17. PMID: 29719953.

[46] Nasrallah IM, Chen YJ, Hsieh MK, Phillips JS, Ternes K, Stockbower GE, Sheline Y, McMillan CT, Grossman M, Wolk DA. 18F-Flortaucipir PET/MRI Correlations in Nonamnestic and Amnestic Variants of Alzheimer Disease. *J Nucl Med.* 2018 Feb;59(2):299-306. doi: 10.2967/jnumed.117.194282. Epub 2017 Jul 26. Erratum in: *J Nucl Med.* 2019 May;60(5):709. PMID: 28747523; PMCID: PMC6348438.

[47] Zhou Y, Bai B. Tau and Pet/Mri Imaging Biomarkers for Detecting and Diagnosing Early Dementia. *Jacobs J Med Diagn Med Imaging.* 2017 Nov;2(1):017. Epub 2017 Aug 8. PMID: 29026896; PMCID: PMC5634528.

[48] Drzezga A, Barthel H, Minoshima S, Sabri O. Potential Clinical Applications of PET/MR Imaging in Neurodegenerative Diseases. *J Nucl Med.* 2014 Jun 1;55(Supplement 2):47S-55S. doi: 10.2967/jnumed.113.129254. Epub 2014 May 12. PMID: 24819417.

[49] Rubí S, Setoain X, Donaire A, Bargalló N, Sanmartí F, Carreño M, Rumià J, Calvo A, Aparicio J, Campistol J, Pons F. Validation of FDG-PET/MRI coregistration in nonlesional refractory childhood epilepsy. *Epilepsia.* 2011 Dec;52(12):2216-24. doi: 10.1111/j.1528-1167.2011.03295.x. Epub 2011 Nov 2. PMID: 22050207.

[50] Leynes AP, Yang J, Wiesinger F, Kaushik SS, Shanbhag DD, Seo Y, Hope TA, Larson PEZ. Zero-Echo-Time and Dixon Deep Pseudo-CT (ZeDD CT): Direct Generation of Pseudo-CT Images for Pelvic PET/MRI Attenuation Correction Using Deep Convolutional Neural Networks with Multiparametric MRI. *J Nucl Med.* 2018 May; 59(5): 852-858. doi: 10.2967/jnumed.117.198051. Epub 2017 Oct 30. PMID: 29084824; PMCID: PMC5932530.

[51] Mehranian A, Arabi H, Zaidi H. Quantitative analysis of MRI-guided attenuation correction techniques in time-of-flight brain

PET/MRI. *Neuroimage.* 2016 Apr 15;130:123-133. doi: 10.1016/j. neuroimage.2016.01.060. Epub 2016 Feb 4. PMID: 26853602.

[52] Tondo G, Esposito M, Dervenoulas G, Wilson H, Politis M, Pagano G. Hybrid PET-MRI Applications in Movement Disorders. *Int Rev Neurobiol.* 2019;144:211-257. doi: 10.1016/bs.irn.2018.10.003. Epub 2018 Nov 8. PMID: 30638455.

[53] Zhou Y. *Imaging and Multiomic Biomarker Applications – Advances in Early Alzheimer's Disease.* Nova Science Publishers. 2020.

[54] Zhou Y. *Multiparametric Imaging in Neurodegenerative Disease.* Nova Science Publishers. 2019.

Chapter 3

FRONTO-TEMPORAL DEMENTIA: IMAGING BIOMARKERS

ABSTRACT

Multiple brain networks were involved in frontotemporal dementia and mainly behavior variant type (bvFTD), that might be related to the brain atrophy and behavioral deficits in patients. The purposes of this work are to: 1. confirm the structural and functional connectivity differences in bvFTD patients using RS-fMRI and DTI data, and apply relatively new VMHC and ICA-DR methods for identifying interhemispheric discoordination and multi-circuit dysregulation in patients; 2. analyze the PET molecular imaging data of FDG glucose-metabolism and amyloid neuropathological burden quantification, and compute the statistical differences between patients and controls with PET data; and 3. compare the differences of RS-fMRI data acquired at several conditions or between groups, including baseline-longitudinal analysis in FTD patients, opening vs. closing eyes conditions for bvFTD together with the conventional bvFTD vs. controls using brain stem as motion restriction.

The advanced MRI and fMRI methods such as VMHC and ICA-DR as well as PET molecular imaging data identified the typical brain atrophy, hypometabolism, neuropathological burden as well as functional dysconnectivity patterns in the orbitofrontal and anterior temporal cortices, with the cerebellum and dorsolateral prefrontal areas as compensation largely. In line with previous work, our MRI/PET results were consistent at multiple levels from molecular, metabolic, functional, structural and microstructural to brain circuits, and added another perspective of comprehensive and multiparametric imaging evidence to the same data cohort.

Keywords: frontotemporal dementia, PET/MRI, behavior variant, dual regression, independent component analysis, voxel-mirrored homotopic correlation, small-worldness, efficiency, glucose metabolism, amyloid accumulation, longitudinal analysis, eyes opening, eyes closing, resting-state fMRI, gray matter atrophy, voxel-based morphometry

1. INTRODUCTION

Frontotemporal dementia (FTD) is a neurodegenerative disorder that has the frontal and temporal lobar abnormalities including atrophy and hypometabolism [1]. The clinical impairments involve multiple domains such as executive function, memory, and emotion; with behavior variant (bv) as one primary type and two variants of primary progressive aphasia (PPA). The bvFTD presents symptom worsening in several aspects including the emotion, social behavior, personal conduct and decision making at a slow pace usually [2]. Decline in attention and executive function together with apathy are the major neurocognitive deficits in FTD patients [3]. Recent diagnosis criteria of possible bvFTD based on DSM-5 include: slow onset and gradual progression of a neurocognitive disorder, as well as at least three behavioral symptoms and a prominent decline in social cognition and/or executive abilities [4]. And the six behavioral symptoms are: a. disinhibition; b. apathy or inertia; c. loss of sympathy or empathy; d. preservative, stereotyped, or compulsive/ritualistic behaviors; e. hyperorality and dietary changes; and f. neuropsychological profile dysexecution such as executive/generation deficits with relative sparing of memory and visuospatial functions [5]. The probable bvFTD meets the criteria of possible bvFTD with additions of significant functional decline and consistent imaging evidence of frontal and/or anterior temporal atrophy or hypometabolism/hypoperfusion [5].

New imaging techniques and modalities including quantitative structural and functional MRI, perfusion and metabolism, neuropathological quantification with PET amyloid and tau tracers have emerged to investigate brain abnormalities in FTD and provide further insight into disease progression across many clinical, genetic and pathological variants [6, 7]. Specifically, the BOLD resting-state (RS)-fMRI signal that is usually acquired with easy clinical set at relatively short time could reveal the functional architecture of the brain with advanced imaging processing methods, including seed-based approaches, independent component analysis, graph theory based small worldness configuration, clustering algorithms, neural network computation, and various pattern recognition based classifiers [8]. Characteristic resting state network (RSN) abnormalities in bvFTD involved not only the salience network (mainly anterior cingulum with both ventral and dorsal portions), but also the default mode network (DMN) and fronto-parietal network (FPN) including dorsolateral prefrontal cortex and precuneus that were associated with attention, inhibition and working memory modulation [9]. For instance, attenuated inter-salience network connectivity including fronto-insular, cingulate, striatal, thalamic and brainstem nodes was found in bvFTD, however with enhanced connectivity within DMN in contrast to the lower DMN found in Alzheimer's disease (AD) [11]. Also the regional connectivity between superior temporal gyrus and cuneal, supracalcarine, intracalcarine cortex and lingual gyrus was decreased in bvFTD [12]. On the other hand, abnormal increased connectivity in several brain networks including the dorsolateral attentional network (DAN) and DMN in bvFTD patients compared to controls were observed, and the changes might be related to decline in executive functions and attention as well as apathy [10].

Furthermore, the salience network functional activity measured with fractional amplitude of low-frequency fluctuation (fALFF), especially the left insula, could predict behavioral changes in FTD patients including the apathy and disinhibition scores [13]. In addition, clinical disease severity correlated with loss of right frontoinsular connectivity and biparietal DMN connectivity enhancement in FTD [10, 14]. Also in bvFTD patients, reduced connectivity in the salience network including the fronto-insular cortex and anterior cingulate were found, together with gray matter atrophy detected in temporal, frontal and parietal regions compared to controls [15]. Additional results identified stereotypy association with the elevated DMN connectivity in the right angular gyrus, and prefrontal hyperconnectivity that might represent a compensatory response for absence of affective feedback during the planning and execution of behavior [16]. And finally, higher affective mentalizing performance in bvFTD were associated with stronger functional connectivity between DMN medial prefrontal node and attentional network as well as increased coherent activity in executive, sensorimotor and fronto-limbic networks, suggesting specific compensatory mechanism for the atrophic changes involving regions of affective mentalizing [17].

Regarding longitudinal differences, connectivity between angular gyrus and right frontoparietal network, as well as between paracingulate gyrus and DMN was lower in bvFTD compared with controls at follow-ups [18]. Furthermore, longitudinal changes with lower connectivity between inferior frontal gyrus and left frontoparietal network were observed in bvFTD patients, compared to the decreased longitudinal precuneus and right frontoparietal network connectivity in Alzheimer's disease (AD). Some relatively novel methods and applications had been reported recently, such as nonlinear factorization, dynamic correlation, and graph theory [19-21]. For instance, by factoring in local and global temporal features of the BOLD signal to capture both linear and non-linear associations, weighted symbolic dependence metric method yielded better identification of resting-state networks including DMN and salience network with higher disease classification accuracy in FTD compared to conventional method [22]. Using relatively new dynamic connectivity computation with independent component analysis and sliding-time window correlation methods, RS-fMRI data presented diminished dynamic fluidity together with less meta-states and shifting in presymptomatic FTD compared to controls [23]. Based on graph theory with EEG data, FTD patients had increased small-worldness with higher local but lower global efficiencies compared to controls, indicating functional reorganization toward a more 'ordered' network structure in patients [24].

In summary, multiple brain networks were involved in bvFTD and might be related to the brain atrophy as well as behavioral deficits in patients. The purposes of this work are to: 1. confirm the structural and functional connectivity differences in bvFTD patients using RS-fMRI and DTI data, and apply relatively new VMHC and ICA-DR methods for identifying interhemispheric dis-coordination and multi-circuit dysregulation in patients; 2. analyze the PET molecular imaging data for FDG-metabolism and amyloid neuropathological burden quantification and compare the differences between patients and controls; and 3. perform these analyses to compare the differences of RS-fMRI data acquired at several conditions including baseline-longitudinal comparison in patients, opening vs. closing eyes conditions for bvFTD in addition to the conventional bvFTD vs. controls difference.

2. METHODS AND DATA

2.1. Participants and Data Acquisitions

MRI/PET Imaging data used in the preparation of this article were obtained from the ADNI database (http://ida.loni.usc.edu). The primary goal of ADNI has been to test whether serial MRI, positron emission tomography (PET), other biological markers, and clinical and neuro-psychological assessment can be combined to measure the progression of mild cognitive impairment (MCI) and early Alzheimer's disease (AD). ADNI is the result of efforts of many co-investigators from a broad range of academic institutions and private corporations, and subjects have been recruited from over 50 sites across the United States and Canada. For up-to- date information, see www.adni-info.org.

All the original imaging data used in this chapter were downloaded from the Frontotemporal Lobar Degeneration Neuroimaging initiative

(NIFD) or FTLDNI center as another featured ADNI center (similar to PPMI center as introduced in previous chapters). Available multimodal MRI/PET imaging data included structural MRI for voxel-based morphometry (VBM), PET FDG glucose metabolism and PiB tracer for amyloid accumulation quantification, MRI diffusion tensor imaging (DTI) data, and resting-state (RS)-fMRI data acquired at multiple conditions. The imaging data of FTD patients (mainly behavior variant-bvFTD subtype) and normal controls (NC) were processed with in-house software. The demographic information including age and gender of participants in each modality and sub-group are listed in Table 1.

Table 1. Demographic information of subjects for four types of imaging modalities in the FTD data cohort, including 1-VBM with MPRAGE data, 2-PET molecular imaging with FDG and amyloid, 3-DTI analysis and 4-6 resting-state (RS)-fMRI data

Group	Age (Years)	Women N/%	Total N
1-VBM - Controls	63.9 ± 2.7	6/75%	8
1-VBM - bvFTD	64.1 ± 1.2	3/23%	13
2-PET-Controls	66.8 ± 2.4	3/60%	5
2-PET- bvFTD	64.5 ± 2.2	1/17%	6
3-DTI - Controls	64.5 ± 3.6	4/67%	6
3-DTI - bvFTD	65.3 ± 1.3	2/25%	8
4-BS RS-fMRI Controls	66.1 ± 1.0	9/100%	9
4-BS RS-fMRI FTD	70.6 ± 3.5	2/25%	8
5-EC FTD (Baseline)	68.2 ± 2.1	8/36%	22
5-EO FTD (Baseline)	64.5 ± 2.2	3/60%	5
6-EC-Longitudinal FTD	68.8 ± 3.5	5/42%	12

In the Resting-state (RS) fMRI, three subtypes of comparisons were performed including comparisons of fMRI data between: a) 4-baseline (BS) FTD and 4-BS normal controls (NC) using brain stem as motion restriction during image acquisition; b) 5-eye closing (EC) and 5- eye opening (EO) relaxing conditions of FTD patients during data acquisition at baseline; and c) 6-longitudinal follow-up (1-3 years) visits and matched subsets data at baseline from 4-BS FTD with eye closing condition for FTD patients.

2.2. Imaging Parameters and Post-Processing

All MRI experiments were performed using the 3T MRI scanner with standardized imaging protocols. The 3D MPRAGE (TR/TE/TI = 2300/900/3.0 ms, flip angle = 9°, matrix size = 240 x 256 x 160, resolution = 1 x 1x 1 mm^3) was obtained for reference image used in RS-fMRI connectivity/conductivity maps, as well as for structural morphological analysis. The gray matter atrophy results were obtained using the FMRIB Software Library (FSL) (www.fmrib.ox.ac.uk/fsl) VBM package with statistical permutation analyses based on 3D-MPRAGE data.

DTI data was obtained with standard spin-echo EPI sequence (TR/TE = 10000/62.3 msec, flip angle = 90°, number of diffusion directions = 41, spatial resolution = 1.4 x 1.4 x 2.7 mm^3). The fractional anisotropy (FA) images were converted from DTI data with dcm2nii software (https://people.cas.sc.edu/roden/mricron/dcm2nii.html), and then analyzed using the FSL tract-based spatial statistics (TBSS) software for group difference. Finally, the PET PiB for amyloid accumulation and FDG data were downloaded and processed with the Analysis of Functional NeuroImages (AFNI) (http://afni.nimh.nih.gov/afni) and FSL packages for realignment and normalization respectively, together with statistical parametric mapping (SPM) (http://fil.ion.ucl.ac.uk/spm) for voxel-wise whole brain comparison with 2nd-level ANOVA post-analysis.

For the resting-state (RS)-fMRI data acquired with eyes closing and eyes opening conditions, a standard gradient-echo EPI sequence (TR/TE = 2000/27 msec, flip angle = 80°, number of volumes = 240, spatial resolution = 2.5 x 2.5 x 3.0 mm^3) was performed. RS-fMRI data for the same patient at follow-up visit during 1-3 years of interval with eyes closing together with baseline scan were used for longitudinal analysis with AFNI paired t-test tool. For the resting-state (RS)-fMRI data acquired with brain stem for motion restriction in both FTD patients and controls at baseline , a standard gradient-echo EPI sequence (TR/TE = 5150/31 msec, flip angle = 90°, number of volumes = 96, isotropic spatial resolution = 2.2 x 2.2 x 2.2 mm^3) was performed. Similar to the methods described in Chapter 1, the RS-fMRI data were preprocessed with motion correction and outlier screening such as mean frame displacement (FD) < 0.6 mm to remove excessive motion. The quantitative VMHC, fALFF and RSFC as well as ICA-DR results were processed and analyzed using the same methods as described in the previous Chapter 1 for Parkinson's disease.

3. RESULTS

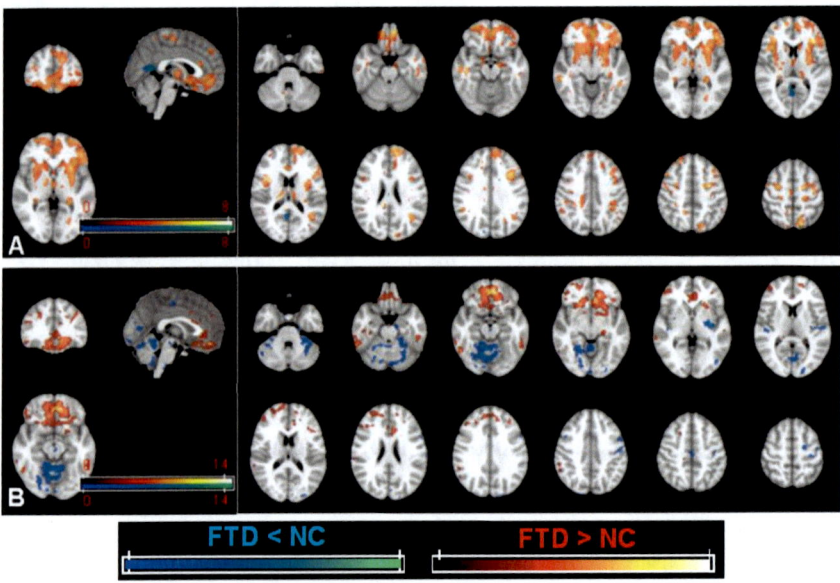

Figure 1. A: VBM showing mostly gray matter atrophy in FTD patients compared to controls (red color); B: PIB amyloid accumulation differences between FTD patients and NC (P < 0.01; blue for FTD<NC and red for FTD>NC). Atrophies in orbitofrontal cortex, scattered temporal regions, medial prefrontal, striatum such as putamen and caudate, insular, motor, premotor, dorsolateral prefrontal cortex, dorsal attentional network including superior parietal region were observed in FTD patients compared to controls (A; red color) as in A. Only a couple of small clusters in the primary visual cortex presented larger gray mater density in patients (A; blue color). Increment of neuropathological amyloid burden measured with PiB tracer were found in regions of temporal and frontal regions (mainly anterior temporal and orbito-medial frontal portion) in FTD compare to NC groups (red in B), accompanied with relatively lower amyloid accumulation in the cerebellum and small clusters in the visual cortex and motor area (blue in B).

Based on structural MPRAGE data analyzed with VBM, mostly brain atrophies in orbitofrontal cortex, scattered temporal regions, medial prefrontal, striatum including putamen and caudate, insular, motor, premotor, dorsolateral prefrontal cortex, dorsal attentional network such as superior frontal and parietal regions were observed in FTD patients compared to normal controls (NC) (Figure 1A, P < 0.01). A few small clusters in the primary visual cortex presented larger gray mater density in patients. Increment of neuropathological amyloid burden measured with PiB tracer were found in regions of temporal and frontal regions in bvFTD patients compared to NC (Figure 1B, P < 0.01), accompanied with relatively lower amyloid level in the cerebellum and small clusters in the visual and motor cortices.

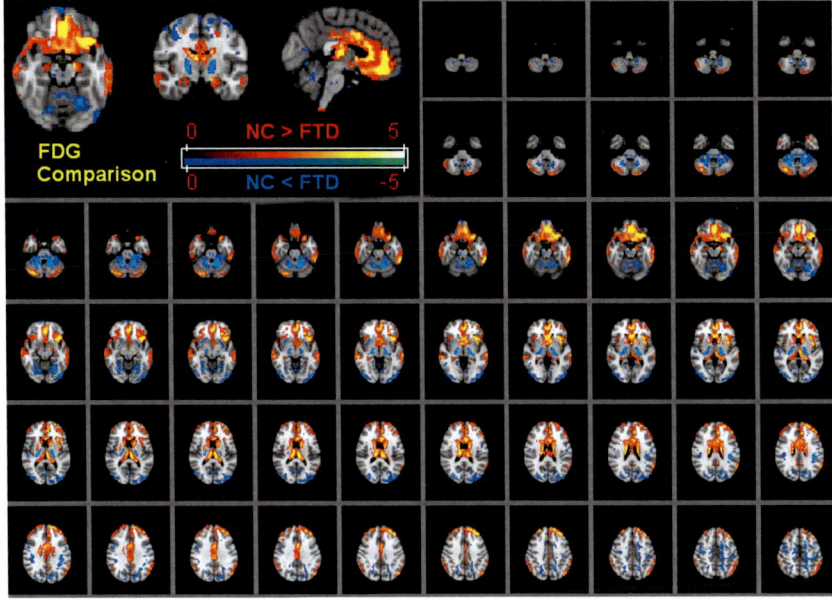

Figure 2. FDG glucose metabolism images comparison between bvFTD and NC demonstrated significant hypometabolism (P < 0.01, red color) in FTD patients in the orbitofrontal cortex, temporal regions including hippocampus and anterior portion, lateral-medial thalamus, anterior and middle cingulate, medial frontal cortex, insular, fronto-parietal and dorsal attentional networks; with higher FDG uptake in the cerebellum, visual cortex, basal ganglia, precuneus and motor areas were observed in patients as well (blue color).

PET FDG glucose hypometabolism in FTD patients in large brain areas including the orbitofrontal and medial prefrontal cortices, temporal regions including amygdala, hippocampus and anterior portion, lateral-medial thalamus, anterior and middle cingulate, insular, fronto-parietal and dorsal attentional networks were identified in bvFTD patients compared to controls (Figure 2; $P<0.01$). In contrast, higher FDG uptake in the cerebellum, visual cortex, basal ganglia, precuneus and motor areas were observed in FTD patients as well. Furthermore, Figure 3 illustrated the white matter TBSS results of FA analysis between FTD and NC with lower FA in the genu of corpus callosum, both limbs of the internal capsule, and small clusters in cerebral peduncle and sagittal striatum (statistical $P < 0.05$; cluster-corrected).

Lower (i.e., worsening) interhemispheric correlation based on VMHC analysis in the inferior parietal and temporal, insular, superior frontal and visual cuneus and calcarine regions as well as cerebellum were identified at longitudinal follow-ups compared to baseline in bvFTD patients (Figure 4A; $P < 0.01$). On the other hand, higher VMHC values existed in the thalamus, motor and supplementary motor cortices, small regions in the temporal cortex including hippocampus and amygdala, periventricular white matter, and superior parietal regions longitudinally. The cross-sectional comparison between FTD patients and controls identified lower VMHC conductivity in temporal, orbitofrontal, visual and parietal cortices in patients (Figure 4B; $P < 0.01$). In contrast, higher conductivity in the cerebellum, dorsolateral attention network, salience network including insular, superior frontal and parietal regions were identified in FTD as well. Finally, significantly lower VMHC in large brain areas in the subcortical caudate, thalamus, hypothalamus, insular, motor/premotor, parietal, visual, frontal and temporal regions such as amygdala and hippocampus were observed in FTD patients for RS-fMRI acquired at opening eyes compared to closing eyes relaxing conditions (Figure 4C; $P < 0.01$).

Only a few small clusters in the unilateral inferior parietal, middle occipital and temporal cortices presented relatively higher coordination in patients, mostly caused by motion artifacts (and possible normalization error) in the VMHC computation, especially in patients with eyes opening.

Furthermore, slightly changes of network functional connectivity at longitudinal follow-ups compared to baseline in bvFTD patients, primarily in the original independent component analysis (ICA) network-seed regions were observed, using inter-network remapping with ICA-DR method (Figure 5; $P < 0.01$).

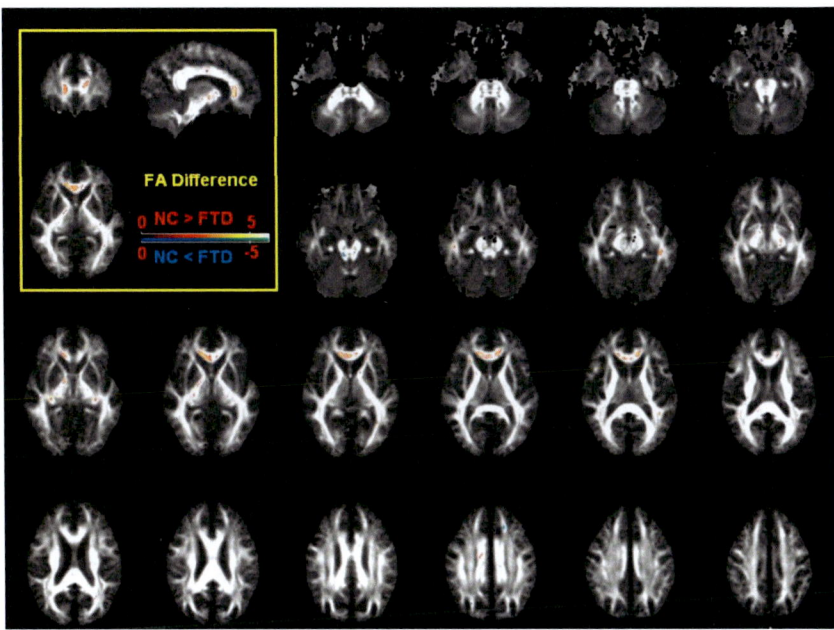

Figure 3. White matter TBSS analysis results of FA between FTD and NC demonstrated lower FA in the genu of corpus callosum, both anterior and posterior limbs of the internal capsule, and small clusters in cerebral peduncle and sagittal striatum in FTD patients (statistical $P < 0.05$; cluster-corrected; red color). A couple of small clusters in the brain stem showed relatively higher FA (blue color) in FTD.

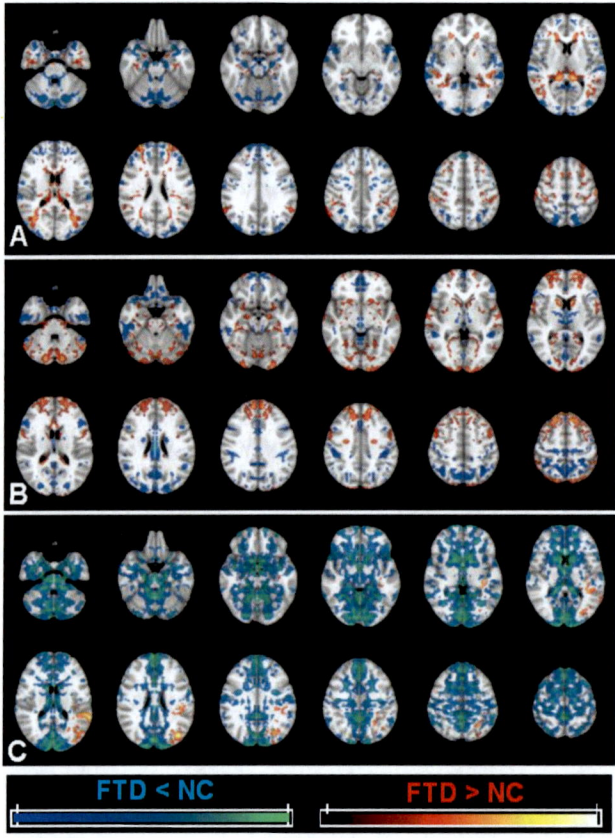

Figure 4. VMHC differences based on RS-fMRI data between A: baseline and longitudinal follow-ups in FTD patients. Lower (worsening) interhemispheric connectivity in the inferior parietal and temporal, insular, superior frontal and visual cuneus and calcarine regions as well as cerebellum were identified at longitudinal follow-ups compared to baseline ($P < 0.01$, blue color). On the contrary, increased conductivity in the thalamus, motor and supplementary motor cortices, small regions in the temporal cortex including hippocampus, periventricular white matter, and superior parietal regions were identified at follow-up times in FTD patients (A; red color). B: FTD patients and normal controls (NC): lower conductivity in temporal, orbitofrontal, visual and parietal cortices in FTD patients compared to NC were found ($P < 0.01$, blue color). On the other hand, higher conductivity in the cerebellum, dorsolateral attention network, salience network including insular, superior frontal and parietal regions were identified in patients as well (red color). C: Lower VMHC in the subcortical caudate, thalamus, hypothalamus, insular, motor/premotor, parietal, visual, frontal and temporal regions were observed in FTD patients at opening compared to closing eyes relaxing conditions (blue color). Small clusters of higher connection in unilateral inferior parietal and superior temporal cortices were observed in patients (red color), probably due to motion artifacts and related normalization error.

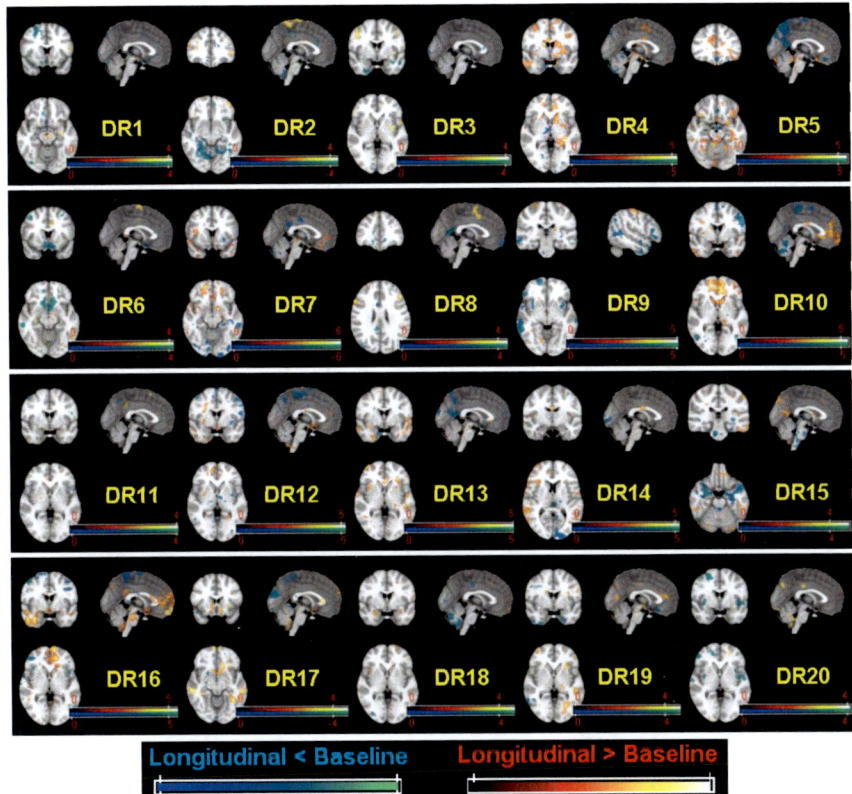

Figure 5. ICA-DR differences between baseline and longitudinal follow-ups (P < 0.01). The longitudinal follow-ups demonstrated slightly changes of network remapping with dual regression methods in the original network-seed regions mainly, compared to baseline in FTD patients. Green-blue for negative longitudinal change (longitudinal < baseline) and orange-red color for positive change in bvFTD group.

In details, decrement of functional intra- and inter- network connectivity at temporal and occipital regions such as fusiform and medial temporal lobe existed in several components including DR2, DR3, DR7 and DR9 (Figure 6A; P < 0.01) at follow-ups compared to baseline. Also decreased orbitofrontal and supplementary motor cortex at follow-ups were found as in DR10, DR6 and DR1, in the temporal regions including hippocampus and medial prefrontal cortex at follow-up compared to baseline as in DR15 and DR16 (Figure 6 A&B; P < 0.01). On the other hand, increased functional connectivity in the cerebellum, superior frontal and motor cortex as in components DRs 3-5 and DR8 were present, together with dorsolateral attentional network and subcortical regions such as hypothalamus and basal ganglia in a few components (Figures 5 & 6).

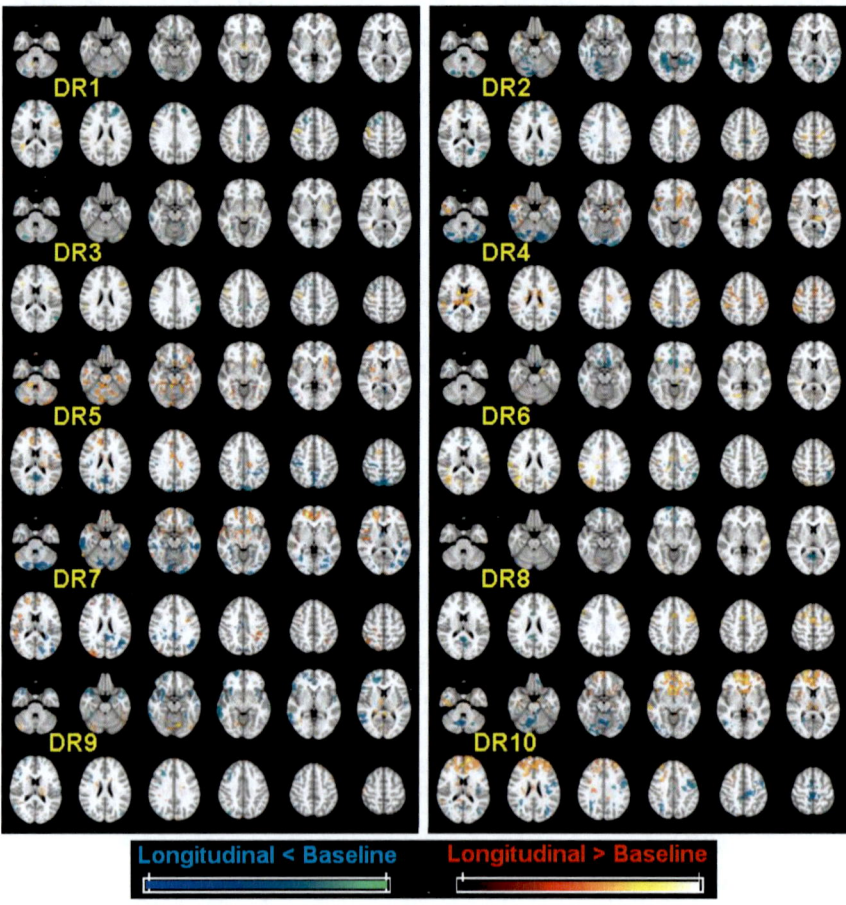

Figure 6A. ICA-DR differences (components 1-10) between baseline and longitudinal follow-ups in multi-slice view of the comparisons (P < 0.01). Decrement of functional connectivity at temporal and occipital regions such as fusiform and medial temporal lobe existed in DR2, DR3, DR7 and DR9 (blue color, P < 0.01) at follow-ups compared to baseline. Also decreased orbitofrontal, supplementary cortex and dorsolateral prefrontal cortex at follow-ups were found as in DR10, DR6 and DR1. On the other hand, increased functional connectivity in the cerebellum, medial frontal and motor cortex as in components DR5, DR 3, DR4 and DR8 were present (red color, P < 0.01).

Fronto-Temporal Dementia: Imaging Biomarkers 81

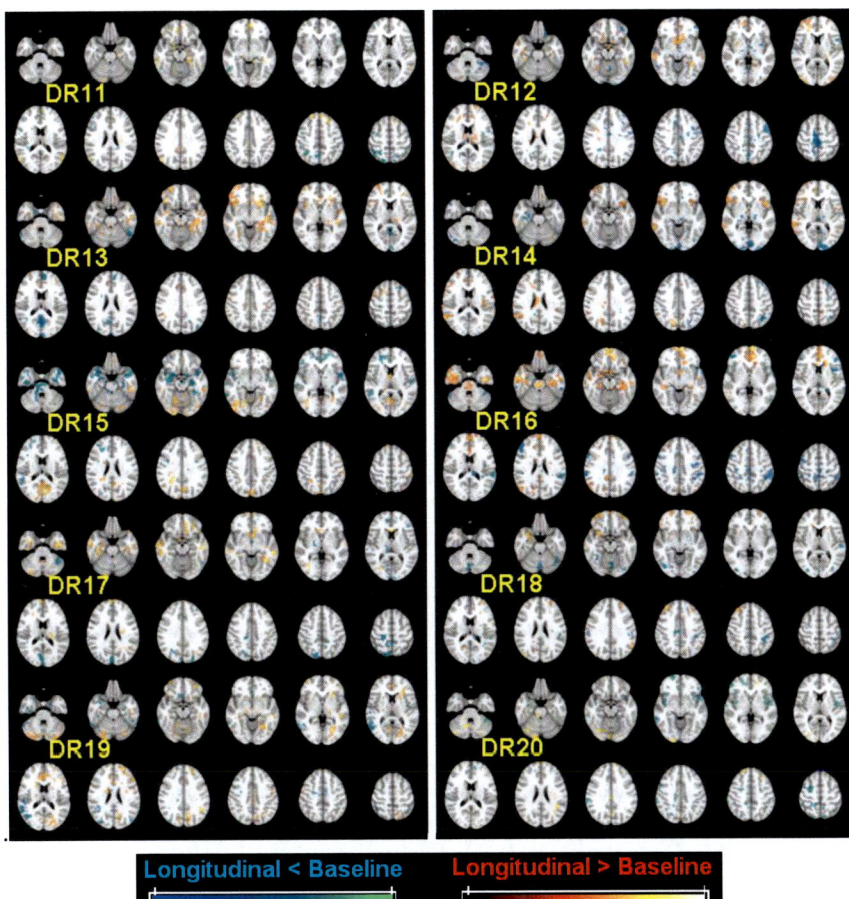

Figure 6B. DR differences (components 11-20) between baseline and longitudinal follow-ups (P < 0.01); blue: 2nd (longitudinal) < 1st (baseline) and red: longitudinal 2nd > 1st visit in patient group. Decreased functional connectivity in the temporal regions including hippocampus, and medial prefrontal cortex at follow-up compared to baseline as in DR15 and DR16 were observed (P < 0.01; blue color). Increased medial prefrontal, anterior temporal, insular, cerebellum and subcortical regions such as hypothalamus and basal ganglia were also observed in most of components (red color).

ICA-DR differences comparing FTD patients to controls with brain stem as the motion restriction identified decrement of functional connectivity at cerebellum, temporal and occipital regions, insular, superior frontal and DMN regions such as posterior cingulate and inferior parietal cortex together with frontoparietal network in majorities of components in Figure 7 largely, and in Figure 8 with multi-slice illustration at significance level of P < 0.01. However, increased connectivity in thalamic network and dorsolateral prefrontal cortex as well as some motor and supplementary motor regions were also observed in patients (Figures 7 & 8, P < 0.01). The statistical differences comparing patients to controls at baseline presented much larger degree of change (spatial size and significance) than the longitudinal differences that were obtained with eyes closing at relatively short interval (1-3 years).

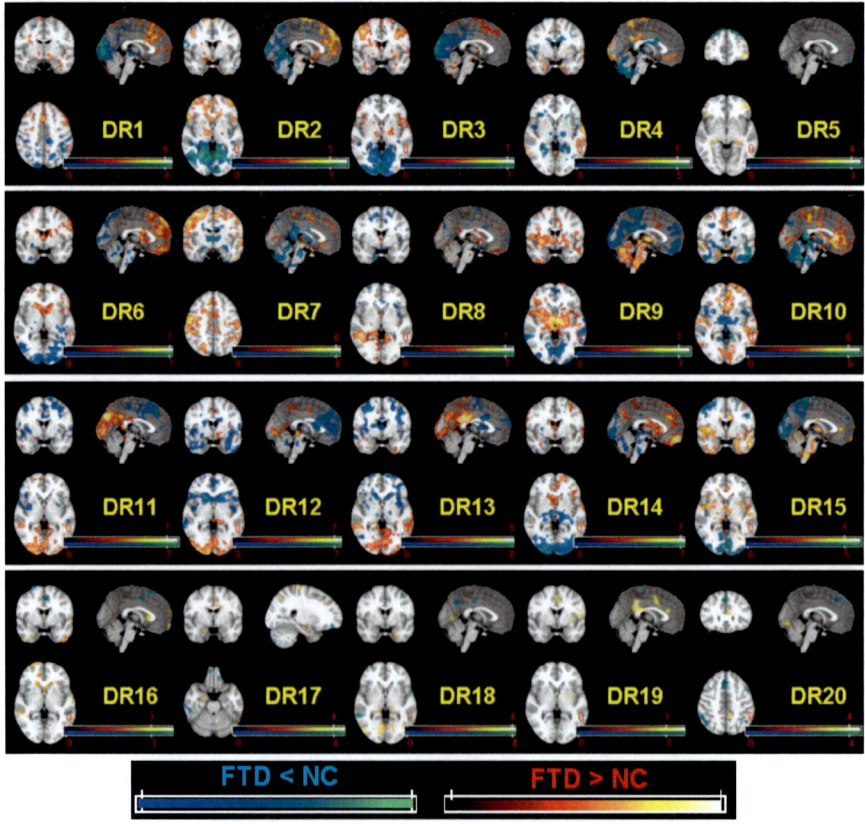

Figure 7. ICA-DR differences between FTD patients and normal controls (NC) (P < 0.01). blue for bvFTD < NC and red for bvFTD > NC for intra- and inter-network connectivity mapping.

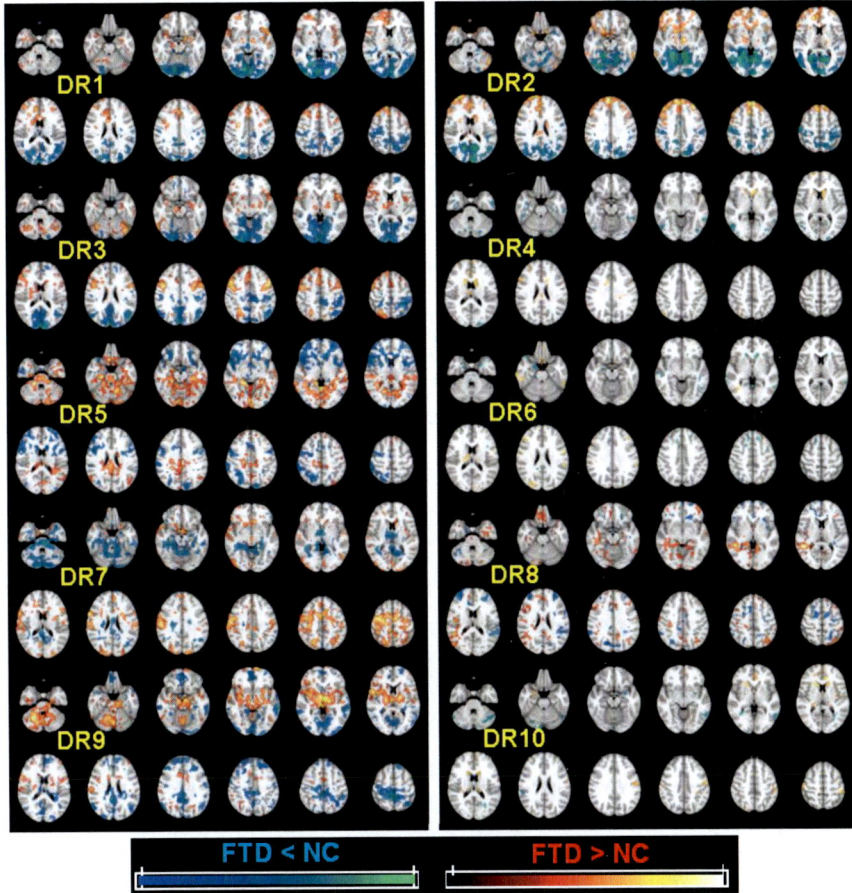

Figure 8A. DR differences (DR components 1-10) between FTD patients and normal controls (NC) ($P < 0.01$). Decrement of functional connectivity at cerebellum, temporal and occipital regions, and DMN regions such as posterior cingulate and inferior parietal cortex, insular and fronto-parietal networks, as well as in motor and supplementary motor cortex were found in majorities of components in FTD patients compared to controls with brain stem as the motion restriction (blue color, $P < 0.01$). On the other hand, increased thalamic and dorsolateral prefrontal cortex as well as some motor and supplementary motor regions were also observed in patients (red color, $P < 0.01$). The statistical differences comparing patients to controls at baseline presented much larger degree (spatial size and significance) than the longitudinal differences at relatively short interval (1-3 years).

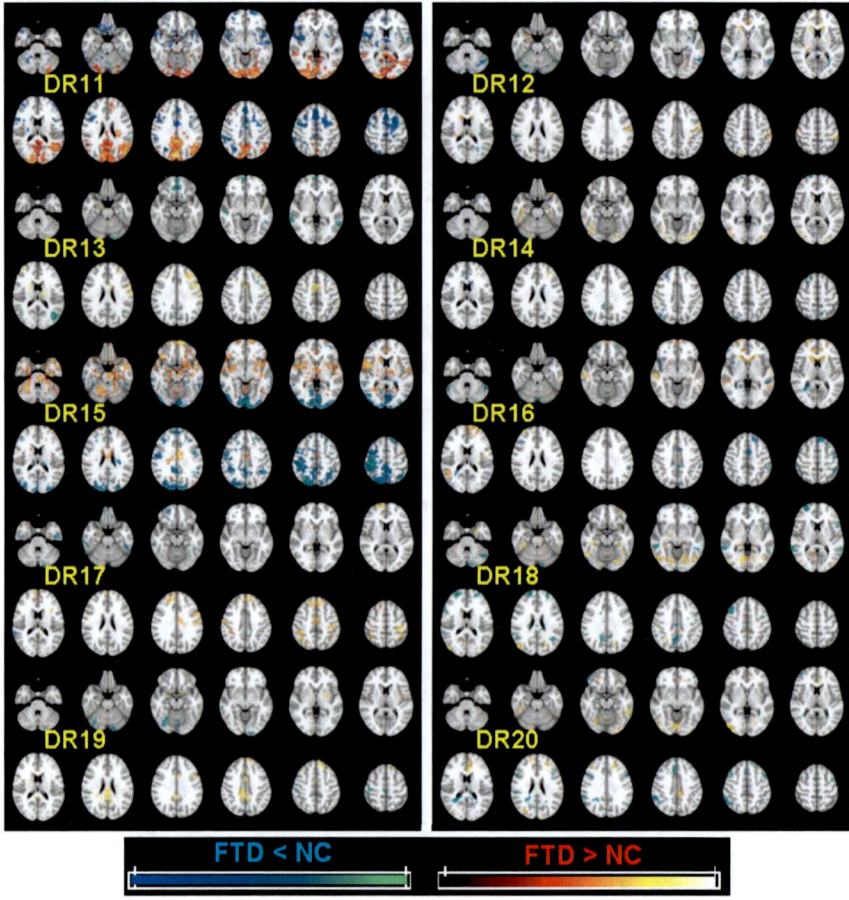

Figure 8B. DR differences (DR components 11-20) between FTD patients and normal controls (NC) ($P < 0.01$); blue for bvFTD < NC and red for bvFTD > NC.

ICA-DR differences of RS-fMRI data comparing opening eyes to closing eyes relaxing conditions in FTD patients found consistent patterns of increased functional connectivity of the inter- DMN and DAN modulation as well as motor/premotor network in contrast to the decreased temporal, visual, insular, fronto-parietal network and striato-thalamo-cortical regions at opening-eyes situation in FTD patients (Figures 9 & 10, majorities of components). These difference regions presented a larger degree of both hyper- and hypo- connectivity pattern compared to the differences between patients and controls using brain stem for motion prevention during RS-fMRI acquisition as in Figures 7 & 8 and much more significant than longitudinal differences in FTD patients as in Figures 5 & 6.

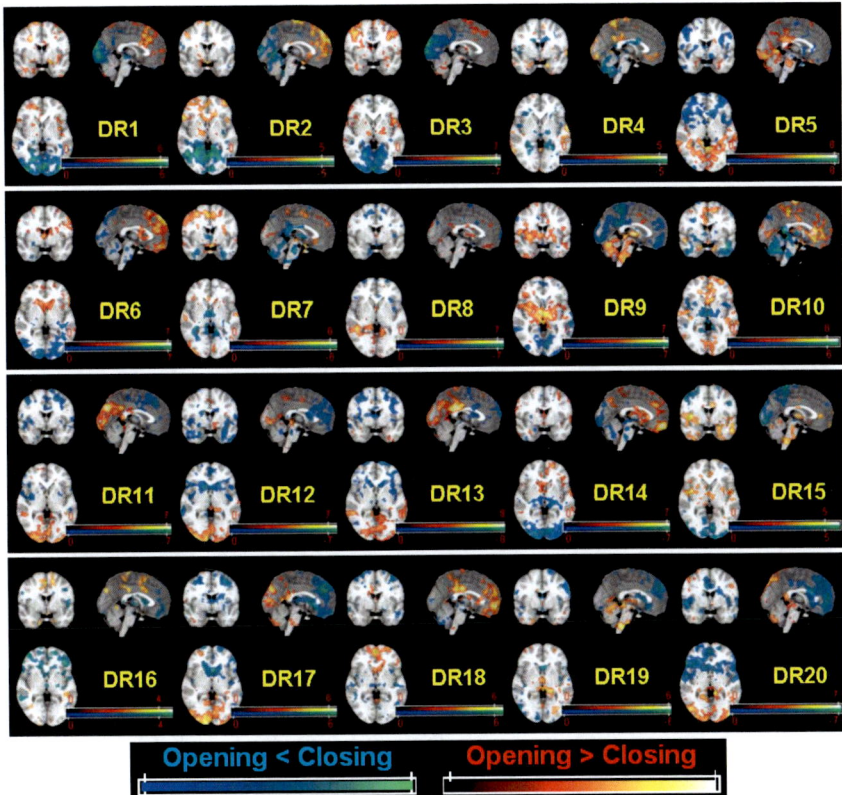

Figure 9. ICA-DR differences of FTD patients between eyes opening and closing relaxing conditions with RS-fMRI data (P < 0.01). Increased functional connectivity in the visual, motor, insular and fronto-parietal networks, dorsolateral prefrontal cortex, DAN and thalamic network were observed in contrast to the decreased temporal, medial prefrontal, inferior parietal and posterior cingulate DMN regions were found at opening eyes compared to closing eyes relaxing condition in FTD patients. These differences regions presented a larger degree of both hyper- and hypo- connectivity compared to the differences between patients and controls using brain stem for motion prevention at RS-fMRI acquisition (Figures 7 & 8) and much larger than longitudinal differences in FTD (Figures 5 & 6). Green-blue for lower and orange-red color for higher functional connectivity in opening compared to closing eyes relaxing condition in FTD patients.

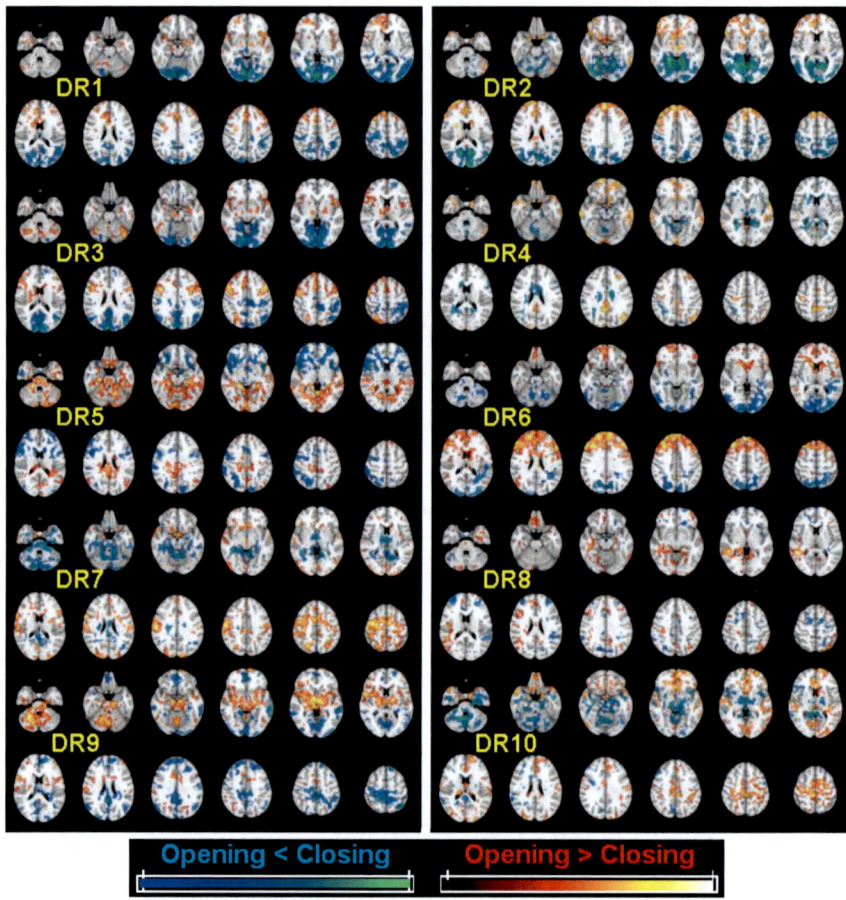

Figure 10A. ICA-DR differences (DR components 1-10) between FTD patients between eyes opening and closing relaxing conditions with RS-fMRI data (P < 0.01); blue: opening < closing eyes and red: opening > closing eyes in bvFTD patients. For instance, decreased functional connectivity in the visual, insular, fronto-parietal network and striato-thalamo-cortical regions were found in multiple components such as DR1, DR4, DR5, DR7-10, DR16, DR17 and DR20 were exhibited. On the other hand, increased inter-DMN and DAN connectivity as well as motor/premotor network in DR2, DR3, DR6, DR11-DR15, DR18 and DR19 were present for probable functional compensation and positive symptoms.

For the network integration, graph theory based small-worldness systematic analysis with the RS-fMRI functional connectivity data were performed and results were in agreement with the VMHC and ICA-DR results. No significant differences of local and global efficiency existed comparing longitudinal to baseline visits within 1-3 years of interval in FTD patients. However, lower relative local efficiency (Gamma) but higher absolute local efficiency (CCFS) were present in FTD patients compared to controls; with higher relative and absolute global efficiencies (Lamda and Lp) in patients (Figure 11).

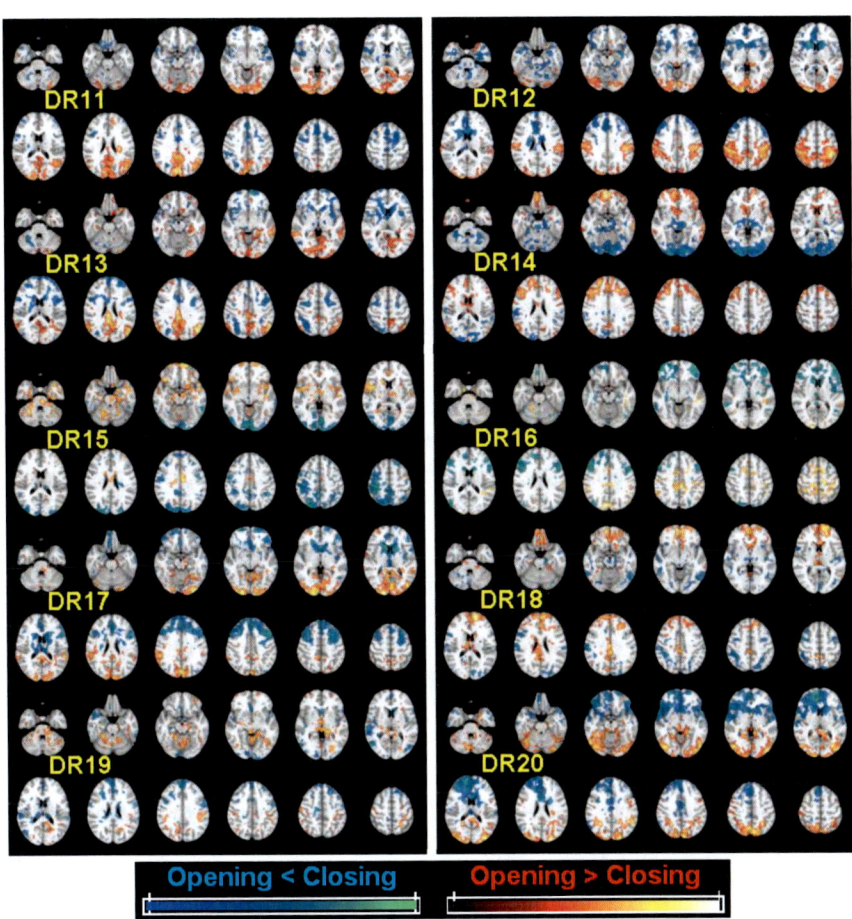

Figure 10B. ICA-DR differences (DR components 11-20) in FTD patients between open eyes and closing eyes relaxing conditions with RS-fMRI data ($P < 0.01$); blue: opening < closing eyes and red: opening > closing eye in patients.

The lower local but higher global efficiency in patients resulted in smaller small-worldness factor (Sigma) in FTD. Furthermore, both absolute local and global efficiencies were largely decreased in FTD patients at eyes opening compared to eyes closing conditions (Figure 12). The small-worldness factor (Sigma) was lower at sparsity level of 0.1-0.12 in eyes opening condition, and was higher when sparsity increased, suggesting the degree of local and global efficiency reductions varied (e.g., higher sigma as expected in the more ordered network topology). Statistical comparisons of mean metrics under two conditions in FTD patients confirmed the quantitative graph differences of opening vs. closing eyes with lower local efficiency of Gamma (P = 0.0018) and CCFS (P = 0.0245), lower absolute global efficiency with longer shortest path length (Lp, P = 0.0029) and altered factor sigma (P = 0.0014) at opening eyes relaxing situation. No other significant differences were found with conventional RSFC, fALFF of whole-band or slow-wave S4/S5 sub-bands quantifications based on the RS-fMRI for either longitudinal comparison, or between FTD and NC groups, or between opening and closing eyes relaxing conditions in patients (P > 0.05).

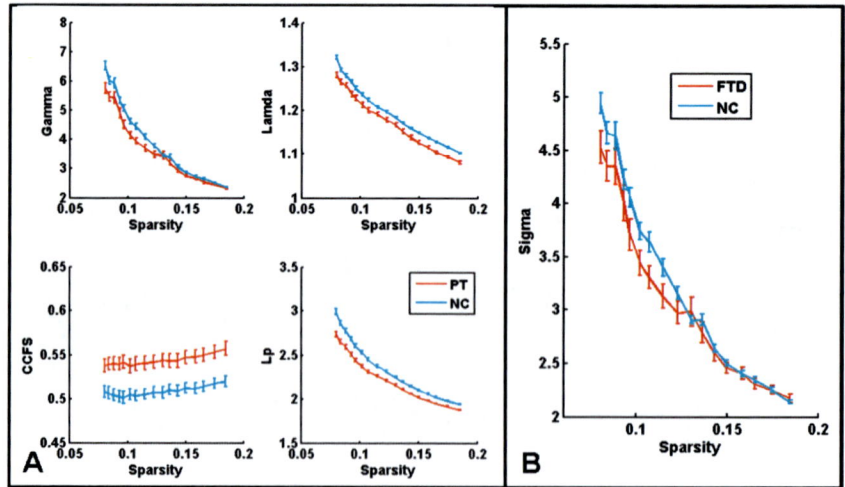

Figure 11. A: Small-worldness based systematic analysis demonstrated lower relative local efficiency (Gamma, red dark line) but higher absolute local efficiency (CCFS) in FTD patients compared to controls (blue light line). Both relative and absolute global efficiencies (Lamda and Lp) were higher (red dark line) in FTD compared to NC with longer shortest path length. B: The scaled small-worldness factor (Sigma) was slightly lower in FTD patients compared to NC, especially at low sparsity level (0.08-0.12).

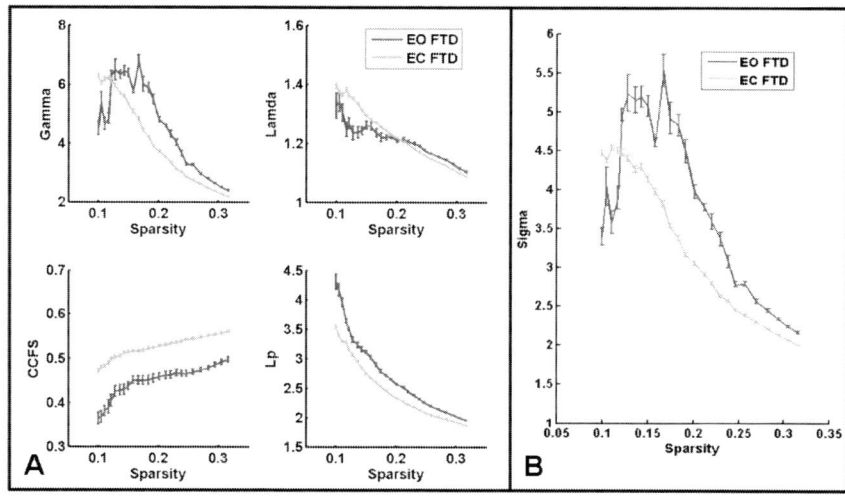

Figure 12. A: Largely decreased absolute local and global efficiencies in FTD patients with eyes opening (EO, red dark line) situation compared to eyes closing (EC, blue light line) situation, in the bottom panel of both CCFS and Lp. B: Small-worldness factor (Sigma) was lower at sparsity level of 0.1-0.12 in EO condition, and was higher when sparsity increased.

4. DISCUSSION

4.1. Summary of Results

Our MRI results of brain atrophy in the frontotemporal regions were in line with the PET molecular imaging results of higher amyloid accumulation and FDG hypometabolism in these regions, especially the orbitofrontal, insular, medial prefrontal and anterior temporal regions. Also the DTI FA identified deteriorated white matter integrity in these regions including genu of corpus callosum and sagittal striatum. Notably, the posterior lateral thalamus also presented atrophy and hypometabolism together with lower FA in the internal capsule including posterior limb. And a few clusters in the hippocampus presented atrophy and hypometabolism as well.

Regarding VMHC conductivity, lower values in the conventional temporal and orbitofrontal cortices were found in FTD patients compared to controls at baseline, as well as worsening at longitudinal follow-up visits (with a less degree compared to cross-sectional comparison). Additional visual and parietal cortices such as calcarine, precuneus and superior parietal lobe also presented lower VMHC in FTD patients at baseline, but some surrounding sub-regions presented higher VMHC at longitudinal comparisons for possible rerouting strategy. On the other hand, higher VMHC values in the cerebellum, primary visual cortex and superior frontal regions comparing FTD to controls at baseline were identified, suggesting compensation roles of these regions that had normal brain reserve without atrophy or hypometabolism at baseline. However, lower values in these regions together with hippocampus and insular were found at longitudinal visit compared to baseline in patients, possibly due to disease progression and injury over time. The subcortical hippocampus, amygdala, caudate and small clusters in the pons had higher VMHC in FTD compared to NC, with lower VMHC in small clusters of basal ganglia such as red nucleus and thalamus. The abnormally higher VMHC in the hippocampus and amygdala at baseline might be related to the disinhibition function in patients, while lower VMHC in thalamus was in line with the hypometabolism and atrophy of these subcortical regions at baseline comparison. Furthermore, in FTD patients comparing opening eyes to closing eyes conditions, largely reduced VMHC values in patients with opening eyes were found in most brain areas including the subcortical regions such as caudate, hippocampus, amygdala, dorso-medial thalamus, hypothalamus and basal ganglia as well as the cortical parietal, primary visual, motor/premotor, insular, medial frontal and anterior temporal regions; indicating more severe deficits at opening eyes relaxing situation in the FTD patients.

As for ICA-based dual regression (ICA-DR) results, consistent with the structural and molecular imaging findings, decrement of functional connectivity at temporal cortex such as hippocampus, fusiform and medial temporal lobe, orbitofrontal and medial prefrontal cortices presented lower fcMRI at longitudinal visit compared to baseline. On the other hand, increased functional connectivity in the cerebellum and dorsolateral attentional network mainly were found as brain circuit rerouting and compensation. ICA-DR differences comparing FTD patients to controls at baseline identified lower functional connectivity in additional DMN regions such as posterior cingulate and inferior parietal cortex, insular and fronto-parietal networks, as well as in motor and supplementary motor cortex, with increased connectivity in the thalamus and dorsolateral prefrontal cortex as well as a few motor and supplementary motor regions. The statistical differences comparing patients to controls at baseline presented much larger degree (both spatial size and significance) than the longitudinal differences that were obtained with eyes closing relaxing condition at relatively short interval (1-3 years). The difference regions comparing opening eyes to closing eyes in patients presented a further larger degree of both hyper- and hypo- connectivity patterns compared to the differences between FTD patients and controls at baseline (such as higher inter- DMN and DAN connectivity) and at a much larger degree than longitudinal differences in FTD patients. The small-worldness analysis confirmed the network integration efficiency alterations in FTD patients with higher global but lower local relative efficiencies compared to NC with less small-worldness factor in FTD at baseline [24]. Furthermore, both local and global efficiencies (especially absolute values) were significantly reduced at opening eyes compared to closing eyes situations in FTD, indicating systematic functional network integration and specialization breakdown in patients at opening eyes relaxing condition.

4.2. Comparison with Previous Findings – MRI/fMRI/DTI/PET Multimodal Results

Atrophy in inferior temporal gyrus, dorsal mid-insula, and hypothalamus was found to be connected to the reduced skin conductance level in patients. Furthermore, the baseline parasympathetic and sympathetic tone was dependent on the integrity of lateralized salience network hubs including the left ventro-anterior insula ROI for parasympathetic function and the right hypothalamus/amygdala regions for sympathetic pathway [25]. Also it had been confirmed that the left-lateralized brain regions in the dominant hemisphere were important for maintaining function of adaptive parasympathetic outflow at baseline [26]. The breakdown of some critical networks including the substantia nigra would impair function of modeling the emotional impact of their own, being apathy and disinhibition for early bvFTD [27]. Also at early stages, the progressive degeneration of the anterior regions of medial frontal structures including atrophy, hypometabolism and/or hypoperfusion characterized the apathy and theory of mind (ToM) deficits of patients [2, 28]. Furthermore, disruption of the fronto-temporal circuit such as the orbitofrontal-amygdala connectivity together with atrophies in these regions including insular in bvFTD suggested relationship between context and sensitive social cognition, also the connection impairments due to deficits in the modeled social context network [29].

Network-based integration analysis found that although globally maintained functional brain architecture, bvFTD patients presented reduced nodal strength in the fronto-insular lobe, altered functional connectivity of fronto-insular and temporal regions and disrupted intrahemispheric connectivity as well [30]. Especially, lowest degree of integration in the thalamus but dysconnectivity in the salience network and subcortical regions with higher global efficiency were observed in patients [31]. Structural covariance of gray matter density using independent component analysis had confirmed the decreased anterior cingulate (i.e., salience) network integrity in bvFTD [32]. Regarding the neurodegeneration consideration, ventricle expansion was prominent at longitudinal one-year follow-up time in bvFTD participants, in addition to the significant atrophy in the frontal lobe, insula, medial and anterior temporal regions bilaterally found at baseline using deformation based morphometry [33].

Using multi-variate pattern analysis (MVPA), the BOLD signal activation differed among the four groups of AD, Parkinson's disease (PD), FTD, and NC in the bilateral inferior temporal gyrus, right central opercular cortex, supramarginal and angular gyri [34]. Also based on multiparametric structural imaging data, reduced cortical thickness in bilateral orbitofrontal and temporal cortex together with lower FA in the corpus callosum, bilateral uncinate fasciculus were identified comparing bvFTD to early onset of AD (EOAD) [35]. Medial prefrontal cortex hypometabolism and hypoperfusion were discovered in FTD compared to controls and AD using PET FDG and MRI arterial spin labeling (ASL) [36]. Moreover, the right prefrontal cortex and bilateral medial frontal lobe demonstrated gray matter atrophy and hypoperfusion, while the premotor cortex presented gray matter atrophy only [37]. Another study confirmed that after accounting for brain atrophy, frontotemporal hypometabolism, particularly in the mesial and orbitofrontal regions existed in the bvFTD group [38].

4.3. Diagnosis Improvement and Future Work

As it had been reported that neuropsychological tests yielded acceptable accuracy for identifying bvFTD from controls, integration of connectivity data such as hypoconnectivity in mid-range frontotemporal links had improved classification power over 90% [39]. Random forest analysis revealed that left inferior parietal cortical thickness (accuracy of 0.78, specificity of 0.76, sensitivity of 0.83) and white matter integrity of the right uncinate fasciculus (accuracy of 0.81, specificity of 0.96, sensitivity of 0.43) were the best predictors of clinical diagnosis [35]. Combining gray matter density (GMD), FA, and RS-fMRI correlations resulted in highest area under curve (AUC) of 0.92 for bvFTD identification from controls [40]. Classification of FTD based on ASL quantification such as hypoperfusion in the anterior cingulate achieved accuracy of 78-85% from controls [41]. An automatic, cross-center and multimodal computational approach for combined imaging information obtained high accuracy (91%), sensitivity (84%), and specificity (97%) for robust classification of bvFTD patients and controls [42].

In line with previous work, our multiparametric imaging results in FTD agreed with each single imaging modality, and displayed expected changes under different conditions [43, 44]. Inclusion of genetics for further disease mechanism, diagnosis and treatment investigation [45-47] as well as applications to other types of FTD such as PPA FTD [48-50] will be some future works.

In conclusion, we had identified the typical brain atrophy, glucose hypometabolism and higher amyloid neuropathological burden, lower interhemispheric correlation and structural connectivity as well as functional intra- and inter- network dysconnectivity patterns in several brain regions including the orbitofrontal and anterior temporal cortices, with the cerebellum and dorsolateral prefrontal areas as compensation in bvFTD patients compared to controls. Moreover, these imaging abnormalities such as lower connectivity and conductivity in insular and fronto-parietal networks but higher inter- DMN and DAN modulation were more severe at opening eyes compared to closing eyes relaxing condition in patients, in contrast to the conventional comparison between bvFTD and NC and least significant in the longitudinal comparison in FTD patients. Our MRI/PET results were consistent and confirmative at multiple levels from molecular, morphological, metabolic, functional, structural and microstructural metrics to brain circuits and systematic integration, and provided further comprehensive and quantitative imaging evidence for better FTD diagnosis, staging and treatment.

REFERENCES

[1] Rohrer JD, Rosen HJ. Neuroimaging in frontotemporal dementia. *Int Rev Psychiatry*. 2013 Apr;25(2):221-9. doi: 10.3109/09540261.2013. 778822. PMID: 23611351.

[2] Seeley WW, Zhou J, Kim EJ. Frontotemporal dementia: what can the behavioral variant teach us about human brain organization? *Neuroscientist*. 2012 Aug;18(4):373-85. doi: 10.1177/1073858 411410354. Epub 2011 Jun 13. PMID: 21670424.

[3] Ducharme S, Price BH, Dickerson BC. Apathy: a neurocircuitry model based on frontotemporal dementia. *J Neurol Neurosurg Psychiatry*. 2018 Apr;89(4):389-396. doi: 10.1136/jnnp-2017-

316277. Epub 2017 Oct 24. PMID: 29066518; PMCID: PMC6561783.

[4] Ducharme S, Price BH, Larvie M, Dougherty DD, Dickerson BC. Clinical Approach to the Differential Diagnosis Between Behavioral Variant Frontotemporal Dementia and Primary Psychiatric Disorders. *Am J Psychiatry.* 2015 Sep 1;172(9):827-37. doi: 10.1176/appi.ajp.2015.14101248. PMID: 26324301.

[5] Rascovsky K, Hodges JR, Knopman D, Mendez MF, Kramer JH, Neuhaus J, van Swieten JC, Seelaar H, Dopper EG, Onyike CU, Hillis AE, Josephs KA, Boeve BF, Kertesz A, Seeley WW, Rankin KP, Johnson JK, Gorno-Tempini ML, Rosen H, Prioleau-Latham CE, Lee A, Kipps CM, Lillo P, Piguet O, Rohrer JD, Rossor MN, Warren JD, Fox NC, Galasko D, Salmon DP, Black SE, Mesulam M, Weintraub S, Dickerson BC, Diehl-Schmid J, Pasquier F, Deramecourt V, Lebert F, Pijnenburg Y, Chow TW, Manes F, Grafman J, Cappa SF, Freedman M, Grossman M, Miller BL. Sensitivity of revised diagnostic criteria for the behavioural variant of frontotemporal dementia. *Brain.* 2011 Sep;134(Pt 9):2456-77. doi: 10.1093/brain/awr179. Epub 2011 Aug 2. PMID: 21810890; PMCID: PMC3170532.

[6] Whitwell JL, Josephs KA. Recent advances in the imaging of frontotemporal dementia. *Curr Neurol Neurosci Rep.* 2012 Dec; 12(6):715-23. doi: 10.1007/s11910-012-0317-0. PMID: 23015371; PMCID: PMC3492940.

[7] Whitwell JL. FTD spectrum: Neuroimaging across the FTD spectrum. *Prog Mol Biol Transl Sci.* 2019;165:187-223. doi: 10.1016/bs.pmbts.2019.05.009. Epub 2019 Jun 18. PMID: 31481163; PMCID: PMC7153045.

[8] Lee MH, Smyser CD, Shimony JS. Resting-state fMRI: a review of methods and clinical applications. *AJNR Am J Neuroradiol.* 2013 Oct;34(10):1866-72. doi: 10.3174/ajnr.A3263. Epub 2012 Aug 30. PMID: 22936095; PMCID: PMC4035703.

[9] Filippi M, Agosta F, Scola E, Canu E, Magnani G, Marcone A, Valsasina P, Caso F, Copetti M, Comi G, Cappa SF, Falini A.

Functional network connectivity in the behavioral variant of frontotemporal dementia. *Cortex.* 2013 Oct;49(9):2389-401. doi: 10.1016/j.cortex.2012.09.017. Epub 2012 Oct 24. PMID: 23164495.

[10] Zhou J, Greicius MD, Gennatas ED, Growdon ME, Jang JY, Rabinovici GD, Kramer JH, Weiner M, Miller BL, Seeley WW. Divergent network connectivity changes in behavioural variant frontotemporal dementia and Alzheimer's disease. *Brain.* 2010 May;133(Pt 5):1352-67. doi: 10.1093/brain/awq075. Epub 2010 Apr 21. PMID: 20410145; PMCID: PMC2912696.

[11] Hafkemeijer A, Möller C, Dopper EG, Jiskoot LC, Schouten TM, van Swieten JC, van der Flier WM, Vrenken H, Pijnenburg YA, Barkhof F, Scheltens P, van der Grond J, Rombouts SA. Resting state functional connectivity differences between behavioral variant frontotemporal dementia and Alzheimer's disease. *Front Hum Neurosci.* 2015 Sep 8;9:474. doi: 10.3389/fnhum.2015.00474. PMID: 26441584; PMCID: PMC4561903.

[12] Rytty R, Nikkinen J, Paavola L, Abou Elseoud A, Moilanen V, Visuri A, Tervonen O, Renton AE, Traynor BJ, Kiviniemi V, Remes AM. GroupICA dual regression analysis of resting state networks in a behavioral variant of frontotemporal dementia. *Front Hum Neurosci.* 2013 Aug 26;7:461. doi: 10.3389/fnhum.2013.00461. PMID: 23986673; PMCID: PMC3752460.

[13] Day GS, Farb NA, Tang-Wai DF, Masellis M, Black SE, Freedman M, Pollock BG, Chow TW. Salience network resting-state activity: prediction of frontotemporal dementia progression. *JAMA Neurol.* 2013 Oct;70(10):1249-53. doi: 10.1001/jamaneurol.2013.3258. PMID: 23959214.

[14] Zhou J, Liu S, Ng KK, Wang J. Applications of Resting-State Functional Connectivity to Neurodegenerative Disease. *Neuroimaging Clin N Am.* 2017 Nov;27(4):663-683. doi: 10.1016/j.nic.2017.06.007. PMID: 28985936.

[15] Farb NA, Grady CL, Strother S, Tang-Wai DF, Masellis M, Black S, Freedman M, Pollock BG, Campbell KL, Hasher L, Chow TW. Abnormal network connectivity in frontotemporal dementia:

evidence for prefrontal isolation. *Cortex.* 2013 Jul-Aug;49(7):1856-73. doi: 10.1016/j.cortex.2012.09.008. Epub 2012 Sep 24. PMID: 23092697.

[16] Farb NA, Grady CL, Strother S, Tang-Wai DF, Masellis M, Black S, Freedman M, Pollock BG, Campbell KL, Hasher L, Chow TW. Abnormal network connectivity in frontotemporal dementia: evidence for prefrontal isolation. *Cortex.* 2013 Jul-Aug;49(7):1856-73. doi: 10.1016/j.cortex.2012.09.008. Epub 2012 Sep 24. PMID: 23092697

[17] Caminiti SP, Canessa N, Cerami C, Dodich A, Crespi C, Iannaccone S, Marcone A, Falini A, Cappa SF. Affective mentalizing and brain activity at rest in the behavioral variant of frontotemporal dementia. *Neuroimage Clin.* 2015 Aug 28;9:484-97. doi: 10.1016/j.nicl.2015.08.012. PMID: 26594631; PMCID: PMC4600858.

[18] Hafkemeijer A, Möller C, Dopper EG, Jiskoot LC, van den Berg-Huysmans AA, van Swieten JC, van der Flier WM, Vrenken H, Pijnenburg YA, Barkhof F, Scheltens P, van der Grond J, Rombouts SA. A Longitudinal Study on Resting State Functional Connectivity in Behavioral Variant Frontotemporal Dementia and Alzheimer's Disease. *J Alzheimers Dis.* 2017;55(2):521-537. doi: 10.3233/JAD-150695. PMID: 27662284.

[19] Banerjee D, Muralidharan A, Hakim Mohammed AR, Malik BH. Neuroimaging in Dementia: A Brief Review. *Cureus.* 2020 Jun 18;12(6):e8682. doi: 10.7759/cureus.8682. PMID: 32699682; PMCID: PMC7370590.

[20] Filippi M, Spinelli EG, Cividini C, Agosta F. Resting State Dynamic Functional Connectivity in Neurodegenerative Conditions: A Review of Magnetic Resonance Imaging Findings. *Front Neurosci.* 2019 Jun 20;13:657. doi: 10.3389/fnins.2019.00657. PMID: 31281241; PMCID: PMC6596427.

[21] Feis RA, Smith SM, Filippini N, Douaud G, Dopper EG, Heise V, Trachtenberg AJ, van Swieten JC, van Buchem MA, Rombouts SA, Mackay CE. ICA-based artifact removal diminishes scan site differences in multi-center resting-state fMRI. *Front Neurosci.* 2015

Oct 27;9:395. doi: 10.3389/fnins.2015.00395. PMID: 26578859; PMCID: PMC4621866.

[22] Moguilner S, García AM, Mikulan E, Hesse E, García-Cordero I, Melloni M, Cervetto S, Serrano C, Herrera E, Reyes P, Matallana D, Manes F, Ibáñez A, Sedeño L. Weighted Symbolic Dependence Metric (wSDM) for fMRI resting-state connectivity: A multicentric validation for frontotemporal dementia. *Sci Rep.* 2018 Jul 25;8(1):11181. doi: 10.1038/s41598-018-29538-9. PMID: 30046142; PMCID: PMC6060104.

[23] Premi E, Calhoun VD, Diano M, Gazzina S, Cosseddu M, Alberici A, Archetti S, Paternicò D, Gasparotti R, van Swieten J, Galimberti D, Sanchez-Valle R, Laforce R Jr, Moreno F, Synofzik M, Graff C, Masellis M, Tartaglia MC, Rowe J, Vandenberghe R, Finger E, Tagliavini F, de Mendonça A, Santana I, Butler C, Ducharme S, Gerhard A, Danek A, Levin J, Otto M, Frisoni G, Cappa S, Sorbi S, Padovani A, Rohrer JD, Borroni B; Genetic FTD Initiative, GENFI. *The inner fluctuations of the brain in presymptomatic Frontotemporal Dementia: The chronnectome fingerprint. Neuroimage.* 2019 Apr 1; 189:645-654. doi: 10.1016/j.neuroimage.2019.01.080. Epub 2019 Feb 1. PMID: 30716457; PMCID: PMC6669888.

[24] de Haan W, Pijnenburg YA, Strijers RL, van der Made Y, van der Flier WM, Scheltens P, Stam CJ. Functional neural network analysis in frontotemporal dementia and Alzheimer's disease using EEG and graph theory. *BMC Neurosci.* 2009 Aug 21;10:101. doi: 10.1186/1471-2202-10-101. PMID: 19698093; PMCID: PMC2736175.

[25] Sturm VE, Brown JA, Hua AY, Lwi SJ, Zhou J, Kurth F, Eickhoff SB, Rosen HJ, Kramer JH, Miller BL, Levenson RW, Seeley WW. Network Architecture Underlying Basal Autonomic Outflow: Evidence from Frontotemporal Dementia. *J Neurosci.* 2018 Oct 17;38(42):8943-8955. doi: 10.1523/JNEUROSCI.0347-18.2018. Epub 2018 Sep 4. PMID: 30181137; PMCID: PMC6191520.

[26] Guo CC, Sturm VE, Zhou J, Gennatas ED, Trujillo AJ, Hua AY, Crawford R, Stables L, Kramer JH, Rankin K, Levenson RW, Rosen

HJ, Miller BL, Seeley WW. Dominant hemisphere lateralization of cortical parasympathetic control as revealed by frontotemporal dementia. *Proc Natl Acad Sci U S A*. 2016 Apr 26;113(17):E2430-9. doi: 10.1073/pnas.1509184113. Epub 2016 Apr 11. Erratum in: Proc Natl Acad Sci U S A. 2016 Jul 5;113(27):E3985. PMID: 27071080; PMCID: PMC4855566.

[27] Seeley WW. Anterior insula degeneration in frontotemporal dementia. *Brain Struct Funct*. 2010 Jun;214(5-6):465-75. doi: 10.1007/s00429-010-0263-z. Epub 2010 May 29. PMID: 20512369; PMCID: PMC2886907.

[28] Adenzato M, Cavallo M, Enrici I. Theory of mind ability in the behavioural variant of frontotemporal dementia: an analysis of the neural, cognitive, and social levels. *Neuropsychologia*. 2010 Jan;48(1):2-12. doi: 10.1016/j.neuropsychologia.2009.08.001. PMID: 19666039.

[29] Ibañez A, Manes F. Contextual social cognition and the behavioral variant of frontotemporal dementia. *Neurology*. 2012 Apr 24;78(17):1354-62. doi: 10.1212/WNL.0b013e3182518375. PMID: 22529204; PMCID: PMC3335455.

[30] Filippi M, Basaia S, Canu E, Imperiale F, Meani A, Caso F, Magnani G, Falautano M, Comi G, Falini A, Agosta F. Brain network connectivity differs in early-onset neurodegenerative dementia. *Neurology*. 2017 Oct 24;89(17):1764-1772. doi: 10.1212/WNL.0000000000004577. Epub 2017 Sep 27. PMID: 28954876; PMCID: PMC5664301.

[31] Ng ASL, Wang J, Ng KK, Chong JSX, Qian X, Lim JKW, Tan YJ, Yong ACW, Chander RJ, Hameed S, Ting SKS, Kandiah N, Zhou JH. Distinct network topology in Alzheimer's disease and behavioral variant frontotemporal dementia. *Alzheimers Res Ther*. 2021 Jan 6;13(1):13. doi: 10.1186/s13195-020-00752-w. PMID: 33407913; PMCID: PMC7786961.

[32] Hafkemeijer A, Möller C, Dopper EG, Jiskoot LC, van den Berg-Huysmans AA, van Swieten JC, van der Flier WM, Vrenken H, Pijnenburg YA, Barkhof F, Scheltens P, van der Grond J, Rombouts

SA. Differences in structural covariance brain networks between behavioral variant frontotemporal dementia and Alzheimer's disease. *Hum Brain Mapp.* 2016 Mar;37(3):978-88. doi: 10.1002/hbm.23081. Epub 2015 Dec 10. PMID: 26660857; PMCID: PMC6867562.

[33] Manera AL, Dadar M, Collins DL, Ducharme S; Frontotemporal Lobar Degeneration Neuroimaging Initiative. Deformation based morphometry study of longitudinal MRI changes in behavioral variant frontotemporal dementia. *Neuroimage Clin.* 2019;24:102079. doi: 10.1016/j.nicl.2019.102079. Epub 2019 Nov 5. PMID: 31795051; PMCID: PMC6879994.

[34] Multani N, Taghdiri F, Anor CJ, Varriano B, Misquitta K, Tang-Wai DF, Keren R, Fox S, Lang AE, Vijverman AC, Marras C, Tartaglia MC. Association Between Social Cognition Changes and Resting State Functional Connectivity in Frontotemporal Dementia, Alzheimer's Disease, Parkinson's Disease, and Healthy Controls. *Front Neurosci.* 2019 Nov 22;13:1259. doi: 10.3389/fnins.2019.01259. PMID: 31824254; PMCID: PMC6883726.

[35] Canu E, Agosta F, Mandic-Stojmenovic G, Stojković T, Stefanova E, Inuggi A, Imperiale F, Copetti M, Kostic VS, Filippi M. Multiparametric MRI to distinguish early onset Alzheimer's disease and behavioural variant of frontotemporal dementia. *Neuroimage Clin.* 2017 May 25;15:428-438. doi: 10.1016/j.nicl.2017.05.018. PMID: 28616383; PMCID: PMC5458769.

[36] Verfaillie SC, Adriaanse SM, Binnewijzend MA, Benedictus MR, Ossenkoppele R, Wattjes MP, Pijnenburg YA, van der Flier WM, Lammertsma AA, Kuijer JP, Boellaard R, Scheltens P, van Berckel BN, Barkhof F. Cerebral perfusion and glucose metabolism in Alzheimer's disease and frontotemporal dementia: two sides of the same coin? *Eur Radiol.* 2015 Oct;25(10):3050-9. doi: 10.1007/s00330-015-3696-1. Epub 2015 Apr 22. PMID: 25899416; PMCID: PMC4562004.

[37] Shimizu S, Zhang Y, Laxamana J, Miller BL, Kramer JH, Weiner MW, Schuff N. Concordance and discordance between brain perfusion and atrophy in frontotemporal dementia. *Brain Imaging*

Behav. 2010 Mar;4(1):46-54. doi: 10.1007/s11682-009-9084-1. PMID: 20503113; PMCID: PMC2854356.

[38] Kipps CM, Hodges JR, Fryer TD, Nestor PJ. Combined magnetic resonance imaging and positron emission tomography brain imaging in behavioural variant frontotemporal degeneration: refining the clinical phenotype. *Brain.* 2009 Sep;132(Pt 9):2566-78. doi: 10.1093/brain/awp077. Epub 2009 May 4. PMID: 19416953.

[39] Dottori M, Sedeño L, Martorell Caro M, Alifano F, Hesse E, Mikulan E, García AM, Ruiz-Tagle A, Lillo P, Slachevsky A, Serrano C, Fraiman D, Ibanez A. Towards affordable biomarkers of frontotemporal dementia: A classification study via network's information sharing. *Sci Rep.* 2017 Jun 19;7(1):3822. doi: 10.1038/s41598-017-04204-8. PMID: 28630492; PMCID: PMC5476568.

[40] Bouts MJRJ, Möller C, Hafkemeijer A, van Swieten JC, Dopper E, van der Flier WM, Vrenken H, Wink AM, Pijnenburg YAL, Scheltens P, Barkhof F, Schouten TM, de Vos F, Feis RA, van der Grond J, de Rooij M, Rombouts SARB. Single Subject Classification of Alzheimer's Disease and Behavioral Variant Frontotemporal Dementia Using Anatomical, Diffusion Tensor, and Resting-State Functional Magnetic Resonance Imaging. *J Alzheimers Dis.* 2018; 62(4):1827-1839. doi: 10.3233/JAD-170893. PMID: 29614652.

[41] Steketee RM, Bron EE, Meijboom R, Houston GC, Klein S, Mutsaerts HJ, Mendez Orellana CP, de Jong FJ, van Swieten JC, van der Lugt A, Smits M. Early-stage differentiation between presenile Alzheimer's disease and frontotemporal dementia using arterial spin labeling MRI. *Eur Radiol.* 2016 Jan;26(1):244-53. doi: 10.1007/s00330-015-3789-x. Epub 2015 May 31. PMID: 26024845; PMCID: PMC4666273.

[42] Donnelly-Kehoe PA, Pascariello GO, García AM, Hodges JR, Miller B, Rosen H, Manes F, Landin-Romero R, Matallana D, Serrano C, Herrera E, Reyes P, Santamaria-Garcia H, Kumfor F, Piguet O, Ibanez A, Sedeño L. Robust automated computational approach for classifying frontotemporal neurodegeneration: Multimodal/multicenter neuroimaging. *Alzheimers Dement (Amst).* 2019 Aug

28;11:588-598. doi: 10.1016/j.dadm.2019.06.002. PMID: 31497638; PMCID: PMC6719282.
[43] Irish M, Piguet O, Hodges JR. Self-projection and the default network in frontotemporal dementia. *Nat Rev Neurol.* 2012 Feb 14;8(3):152-61. doi: 10.1038/nrneurol.2012.11. PMID: 22331029.
[44] Filippi M, Agosta F, Ferraro PM. Charting Frontotemporal Dementia: From Genes to Networks. *J Neuroimaging.* 2016 Jan-Feb;26(1):16-27. doi: 10.1111/jon.12316. Epub 2015 Nov 29. PMID: 26617288.
[45] Ishii K. Diagnostic imaging of dementia with Lewy bodies, frontotemporal lobar degeneration, and normal pressure hydrocephalus. *Jpn J Radiol.* 2020 Jan;38(1):64-76. doi: 10.1007/s11604-019-00881-9. Epub 2019 Sep 23. PMID: 31549279.
[46] Greaves CV, Rohrer JD. An update on genetic frontotemporal dementia. *J Neurol.* 2019 Aug;266(8):2075-2086. doi: 10.1007/s00415-019-09363-4. Epub 2019 May 22. PMID: 31119452; PMCID: PMC6647117.
[47] Mutsaerts HJMM, Mirza SS, Petr J, Thomas DL, Cash DM, Bocchetta M, de Vita E, Metcalfe AWS, Shirzadi Z, Robertson AD, Tartaglia MC, Mitchell SB, Black SE, Freedman M, Tang-Wai D, Keren R, Rogaeva E, van Swieten J, Laforce R, Tagliavini F, Borroni B, Galimberti D, Rowe JB, Graff C, Frisoni GB, Finger E, Sorbi S, de Mendonça A, Rohrer JD, MacIntosh BJ, Masellis M; GENetic Frontotemporal dementia Initiative (GENFI). Cerebral perfusion changes in presymptomatic genetic frontotemporal dementia: a GENFI study. Brain. 2019 Apr 1;142(4):1108-1120. doi: 10.1093/brain/awz039. *Erratum in: Brain.* 2019 Jun 1;142(6):e28. PMID: 30847466; PMCID: PMC6439322.
[48] Whitwell JL, Avula R, Master A, Vemuri P, Senjem ML, Jones DT, Jack CR Jr, Josephs KA. Disrupted thalamocortical connectivity in PSP: a resting-state fMRI, DTI, and VBM study. *Parkinsonism Relat Disord.* 2011 Sep;17(8):599-605. doi: 10.1016/j.parkreldis.2011.05.013. Epub 2011 Jun 12. PMID: 21665514; PMCID: PMC3168952.

[49] Meijboom R, Steketee RME, de Koning I, Osse RJ, Jiskoot LC, de Jong FJ, van der Lugt A, van Swieten JC, Smits M. Functional connectivity and microstructural white matter changes in phenocopy frontotemporal dementia. *Eur Radiol.* 2017 Apr;27(4):1352-1360. doi: 10.1007/s00330-016-4490-4. Epub 2016 Jul 19. PMID: 27436017; PMCID: PMC5334426.

[50] Reyes P, Ortega-Merchan MP, Rueda A, Uriza F, Santamaria-García H, Rojas-Serrano N, Rodriguez-Santos J, Velasco-Leon MC, Rodriguez-Parra JD, Mora-Diaz DE, Matallana D. Functional Connectivity Changes in Behavioral, Semantic, and Nonfluent Variants of Frontotemporal Dementia. *Behav Neurol.* 2018 Apr 1; 2018: 9684129. doi: 10.1155/2018/9684129. PMID: 29808100; PMCID: PMC5902123.

Chapter 4

VASCULAR DEMENTIA: BRAIN STRUCTURE AND FUNCTION EVIDENCE

ABSTRACT

Exploring the mechanisms of small vessel disease, especially the relatively severe case of vascular dementia (VaD, higher risks in dependent living participants compared to independent living), and reveal the effects of dependent living (in contrast to independent VaD participants) on the brain are one of the purposes of this study. Utilization of advanced imaging technique including relatively new tract-based white matter microstructural quantification and various diffusivity metrics as well as brain morphology and functional investigation at multiple levels, neural circuits and longitudinal visits is another goal.

Our multiparametric imaging results demonstrated both structural and functional abnormalities in the dependent group compared to independent participants in the VaD data cohort, including lower FA, lower VMHC, brain atrophy and functional connectivity deficits in these patients. Increased global mean neuronal activity with higher fALFF in the slow-wave band S4 and conventional low frequency band (0.01-0.08Hz) together with less efficiency of systematic integration (i.e., lower global but higher local efficiency) based on small-worldness analysis were also exhibited in dependent group compared to independent group. Furthermore, longitudinal changes of FA and diffusivity metrics together with alterations at each visit between two groups in certain brain tracts including cingulum, corticospinal tract and uncinate fasciculus for memory, movement and inhibition connectivity were present, suggesting white matter integrity damage such as demyelination, axonal and Wallerian degeneration in the dependent group. In addition to the agreement of each imaging finding, our systematic and relatively new results could provide neuropathological and neurophysiological clues to the disease severity in general VaD.

Keywords: vascular dementia, dependent living, disability, white matter injury, diffusion tensor imaging, fractional anisotropy, demyelination, axonal degeneration, voxel-mirrored homotopic correlation, fractional amplitude of low frequency fluctuation, slow-wave, small-worldness analysis, efficiency, longitudinal analysis, gray matter atrophy, voxel-based morphometry, tract-based spatial statistics, Wallerian degeneration, corticospinal tract, cingulum, uncinate fasciculus, inferior fronto-occipital fasciculus, corpus callosum

1. INTRODUCTION

The caregiver burden, measured with Zarit Burden Interview (ZBI) instrument score, was significantly higher for patients with abnormal perfusion compared to those with normal perfusion in the bilateral frontal, right parietal and temporal lobes [1]. The behavioral variant frontotemporal dementia (bvFTD) is particularly linked with higher caregiver burden, and Parkinson's disease dementia needs some as well. Cerebral small vessel disease (SVD) is a leading cause of stroke that is a major source of morbidity and mortality in aging population [2]. And stroke is reported to be a major cause of death (ranked 3rd) and long-term disability across the globe, with about half proportion of stroke survivors experience long-term dependency [2, 3]. The neuropathological mechanism underlying SVD, and diagnostic criteria for several subtypes including the vascular cognitive disorder (VCD), vascular dementia (VaD) with neurovascular dysfunction have been investigated extensively [4, 5].

Cerebral vasculature alterations including those affecting the subcortical white matter (WM) microcirculation, might contribute to the cognitive impairment, commonly observed in Alzheimer's disease and stroke [6, 7]. It is expected that diffuse WM abnormalities reflecting loss of myelin and axonal degeneration is one of the imaging hallmarks of VaD, and atrophy of the medial temporal lobe including hippocampus with sclerosis is another feature of VaD [8]. Specifically, the associations of WM hyperintensities (WMH) with stroke, amyloid and fMRI resting state connectivity had been reported previously [9, 10]. Also the vascular reactivity impairment related to multiple sclerosis, disability and depressive symptoms had been found as well [11, 12]. Based on neuroimaging studies, structural changes such as reduced gray matter density in the left striatum and hippocampus, with more frontal WM lesion quantified with WMH images were found in preclinical VaD [13]. In addition, the right lateral prefrontal cortex and left inferior frontopolar regions were involved in both structural and functional imaging deficits [14]. Moreover, the reduced frequency-specific connectivity of the prefrontal cortex, compensated with hyper-synchrony of connectivity among supplementary motor area (SMA) and motor regions might contribute to the disruption of behavioral control such as disinhibition [15]. Studies also reported that distinct regions on the medial wall of the right frontal lobe regulated different behaviors; for instance, apathy was independently associated with tissue loss in the right superior frontal gyrus (SFG). And disinhibition was connected with tissue loss in the right subgenual cingulate gyrus in the ventro-medial prefrontal cortex, while aberrant motor behavior was related to tissue loss in the right dorsal anterior cingulate and left premotor cortex [16].

Further, it was found that the WM fractional anisotropy (FA) measured with MRI diffusion tensor imaging (DTI) of uncinate fasciculus, fibers connecting the frontal and temporal lobes, was correlated with the Hayling test scores for inhibitory functioning [17]. Diffusion MRI, reflecting WM integrity and tissue microenvironment by measuring water molecular movement at multiple directions, adds another perspective by quantifying demyelination and axonal degeneration damage to WM and is more sensitive to tissue microstructural injury than conventional methods [18]. With advanced imaging techniques, the connections between DTI diffusion alterations and the free water in the extracellular fluid compartment space had been modeled and reported [19]. In parallel with the diffusional change, the perfusion volume fraction was increased (could be detected with blood flow or functional T2*-weighted MRI metrics) in the intravoxel motion, and both diffusion/perfusion were related to disease severity [20]. Finally, based on the WM abnormalities detected with DTI, disability was an important causal factor for depression in stroke patients without SVD [21]. With the newly developed advanced WM quantification methods, the correlations between the DTI structural network as well as microstructural extracellular water and cognitive impairment had been reported in SVD and VaD patients [22-24].

Exploring the mechanisms of SVD, especially the relatively severe case of VaD (higher risks in dependent living compared to independent living groups), and revealing the effects of dependent living (in contrast to independent VaD participants) on the brain is one of the purposes of this study. Utilization of advanced imaging technique including relatively new tract-based WM microstructural quantification and various diffusivity metrics as well as brain morphology and functional investigation at multiple levels including neural circuits, systematic analysis and longitudinal visits is another goal.

2. METHODS AND DATA

2.1. Participants and Data Acquisitions

MRI/PET Imaging data used in the preparation of this article were obtained from the ADNI database (http://ida.loni.usc.edu). The primary goal of ADNI has been to test whether serial MRI, positron emission tomography (PET), other biological markers, and clinical and neuropsychological assessment can be combined to measure the progression of mild cognitive impairment (MCI) and early Alzheimer's disease (AD). ADNI is the result of efforts of many co-investigators from a broad range of academic institutions and private corporations, and subjects have been recruited from over 50 sites across the United States and Canada. For up-to-date information, see www.adni-info.org.

One of the ADNI collaborative effort center, the featured Aging Brain with Vasculature, Ischemia and Behavior (ABVIB) project assessed evidence for several possible pathways whereby vascular risk and cerebrovascular disease might adversely impact brain structure and function. All the imaging data used in this chapter were downloaded from the ABVIB center with approval and processed with in-house software. The demographic information including age and gender of participants of each sub-type are listed in Table 1.

Table 1. Demographic information of subjects in two sub-groups (independent vs. dependent groups) of the VaD data cohort

Group	Age (Years)	Women /%(N)	Total N	Dependence Level (1-4)
Independent	77.7 ± 1.0	17/49%	35	1.0 ± 0.0
Dependent	78.7 ± 2.3	3/43%	7	2.3 ± 0.3

The dependence level of participants was assessed with four scales: 1 = Able to live independently, 2 = Requires some assistance with complex activities, 3 = Requires some assistance with basic activities, and 4 = Completely dependent. The range of dependence level for the dependent group was [2-3], with two participants having levels of 2 initially and then were recovered.

2.2. Imaging Parameters and Post-Processing

Available multimodal MRI/PET imaging data included structural MRI for voxel-based morphometry (VBM) analysis and diffusion tensor imaging (DTI) data at both baseline and 2nd visits for cross-sectional and longitudinal comparison. All MRI experiments were performed using the 3T MRI scanner with standardized imaging protocols. For the resting-state (RS)-fMRI data, a standard gradient-echo EPI sequence (TR/TE = 3000/30 msec, flip angle = 90°, number of volumes = 160, spatial resolution = 3.3 x 3.3 x 3.3 mm^3) was performed. The 3D MPRAGE (TR/TE/TI = 2500/1100/3 ms, flip angle = 7°, matrix size = 256 x 256 x 192, resolution = 1 x 1x 1 mm^3) was also obtained for reference image and gray matter atrophy quantification with VBM. DTI data was obtained with standard spin-echo EPI sequence (TR/TE = 9000/101 msec, flip angle = 90°, number of diffusion directions = 65, spatial resolution = 2 x 2 x 2 mm^3).

Resting-state (RS)-fMRI data were processed with similar methods as described in previous chapters to derive VMHC, ICA-dual regression (DR) components, fALFF and conventional seed-based functional connectivity maps in the standard MNI space. fALFF differences between two groups at additional low frequency sub-bands including slow-waves of S5 (0.01-0.027 Hz) and S4 (0.027-0.073 Hz), together with conventional low frequency (LF) of 0.01-0.08Hz were also performed to investigate the neural activity changes. Graph theory based small-worldness analysis was further performed on the preprocessed fMRI correlational data to investigate whole-brain functional network integration and specialization in two groups.

DTI data were first pre-processed with the Diffusion Toolkit toolbox (http://tractvis.org) to obtain the FA and three diffusivity metrics such as axial diffusivity (AD), radial diffusivity (RD) and mean diffusivity (MD) values in original B0 space. For the FA/RD/AD/MD quantification, the FMRIB, Software Library (FSL, http://fsl.fmrib.ox.ac.uk/fsl) tract-based spatial statistics (TBSS) toolbox steps 1–2 (i.e. preprocessing, brain mask extraction with FA > 0.05 and normalization) were used for registration of all participants' FA into the FSL 1-mm white matter skeleton template. The transformation of the individual FA data to the FSL Montreal Neurological Institute (MNI) common space at 1-mm isotropic resolution were implemented with the nonlinear registration tool FNIRT based on a b-spline representation of the registration warp field. After normalization of FA map to the MNI space, tract-specific mean FA values were obtained in 20 main tracts from the well-defined probabilistic tract template (FSL/JHU ICBM atlas). These 20 tracts included bilateral anterior thalamic radiation, corticospinal tract, cingulum, cingulum (for hippocampus connection), inferior fronto-occipital fasciculus, inferior longitudinal fasciculus, superior longitudinal fasciculus (SLF), superior longitudinal fasciculus (temporal part), uncinate fasciculus, and forceps major as well as forceps minor. Quantitative AD/RD/MD values were obtained by applying the same transformation as from individual FA to the template space, and computed with tract-specific mean values [25].

Comparisons between independent and dependent groups were performed at both initial and most recent visits for the DTI data. Longitudinal differences of each sub-group were quantified to the multiple imaging data, including DTI FA and AD/RD/MD diffusivity images as well as tract-based ROI values.

3. RESULTS

The structural atrophy, diffusivity increment and white matter integrity deterioration in a representative vascular dementia patient with MRI T2, T1, and DTI MD, AD and FA metrics were demonstrated in Figure 1.

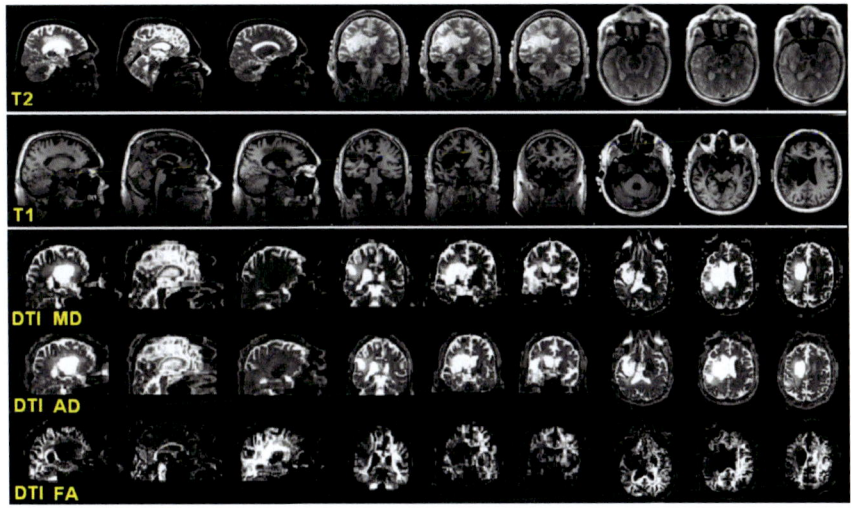

Figure 1. Demonstrative structural atrophy, diffusivity increment and white matter integrity deterioration in a representative vascular dementia patient with MRI T2, T1, and DTI MD, AD and FA metrics.

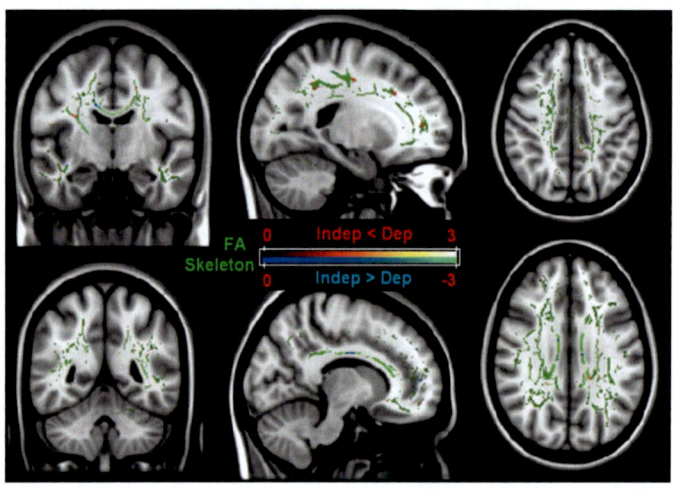

Figure 2. Lower FA values in the corpus callosum (blue color) with altered and some slightly higher FA (red color) in scattered tracts of the superior longitudinal fasciculus, corticospinal tract, uncinate fasciculus and cingulum regions were found in dependent compared to independent participants ($P < 0.05$) based on TBSS. Largely disconnected white matter skeleton (green color) were found, especially for the dependent participants, in the areas of cingulum, cortico-spinal tract, fronto-occipital fasciculus and corpus callosum at even low threshold of FA>0.05 for skeleton projection.

Between-group TBSS analysis using DTI data identified lower FA values in the corpus callosum and altered FA values in scattered tracts such as the superior longitudinal fasciculus, corticospinal tract, uncinate fasciculus and cingulum in dependent group compared to independent participants ($P < 0.05$) (Figure 2). Disconnected white matter bundle on the skeleton were found based on the group mean FA data, especially for the dependent participants, in the areas of cingulum bundle, corticospinal tract, superior longitudinal fasciculus and corpus callosum.

VBM showed gray matter atrophy in dependent participants in the areas of orbitofrontal, temporal, medial frontal, superior frontal gyrus and middle occipital cortices (Figure 3A, $P < 0.05$). While subcortical thalamus, middle cingulate, postcentral sensory, motor and pons areas had higher gray matter density; similar as the hyperintensity of lesions in white matter and subcortical areas with relatively hypointensity on T1 that resulted in higher gray matter density in these regions in dependent compared to independent living participants. Slightly stringent threshold at

P < 0.01 found less regions with only small clusters in fronto-parietal lobe showing atrophy but higher gray matter density in a few subcortical and basal ganglia regions as well as the middle cingulum (Figure 3B, P < 0.01).

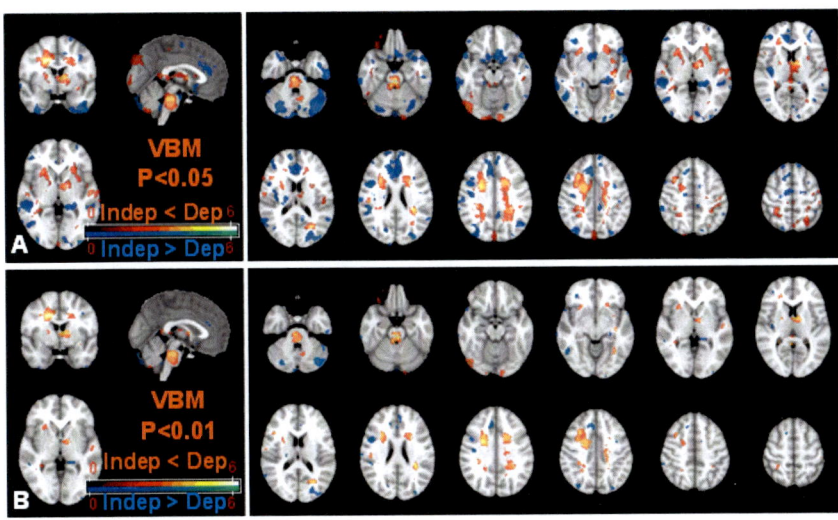

Figure 3. VBM showed gray matter atrophy in the areas of orbitofrontal, temporal, medial frontal, superior frontal gyrus and middle occipital cortices in dependent compared to independent groups (blue color; A: P < 0.05). While subcortical thalamus, middle cingulate, postcentral sensory and motor and pons areas had higher gray matter density in dependent participants (red color in A). Slightly stringent threshold at P < 0.01 found less regions with only small clusters in fronto-parietal area showing atrophy but higher gray matter density in small regions of subcortical and basal ganglia as well as the middle cingulum in dependent group.

Table 2. Brain clusters showing significantly lower VMHC comparing dependent group to independent participants with P < 0.001

Brain Clusters	Cluster Size	P-value	MAX Z score	MAX X(vox)	MAX Y(vox)	MAX Z(vox)
Brain Stem	22087	< 1.0E-34	12.8	44	44	5
Front Pole	481	3.0E-07	9.92	44	94	26
Occipital-Parietal Lobe	249	0.00016	6.69	65	32	56
Somatosensory cortex	195	0.00088	6.38	13	52	48

All brain clusters (size ≥ 195 voxel numbers, maximal Z-score ≥ 6.38) were bilateral for symmetrical VMHC computation.

Figure 4 demonstrated VMHC results with lower interhemispheric coordination in the dependent group compared to independent living participants with P < 0.001 in A and P < 0.01 in B respectively. Monotonically and dramatically decreased VMHC values were found in large brain areas in dependent compared to independent participants, including regions of inferior parietal, dorsolateral prefrontal and orbital frontal cortices such as the triangularis and opercularis regions, frontal pole, basal ganglia including substantia nigra, amygdala and superior frontal cortex, hypothalamus, thalamus, cerebellum, anterior temporal cortex, posterior cingulate, motor area and visual cortex. Lower functional coordination in these areas might reflect language, movement, executive function, memory and visual disabilities. Large cluster size (>190 voxel numbers) with significantly lower VMHC (P < 0.001) in dependent compared to independent groups are listed in Table 2, including brain stem, frontal pole, inferior parietal and lateral occipital lobe as well as somatosensory cortex.

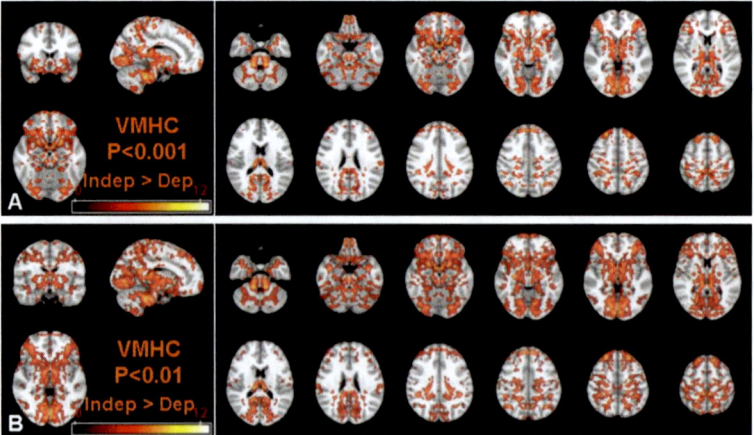

Figure 4. Lower interhemispheric coordination in the dependence living compared to independent living participants with P < 0.001 in A and P < 0.01 in B. Regions of inferior parietal, dorsolateral prefrontal and orbital frontal cortices including the triangularis and opercularis regions, basal ganglia, thalamus, cerebellum, anterior temporal cortex, motor area and visual cortex demonstrated lower coordination that might reflect either language, movement or visual disabilities at high vascular dementia risks and possible more severe case such as stroke.

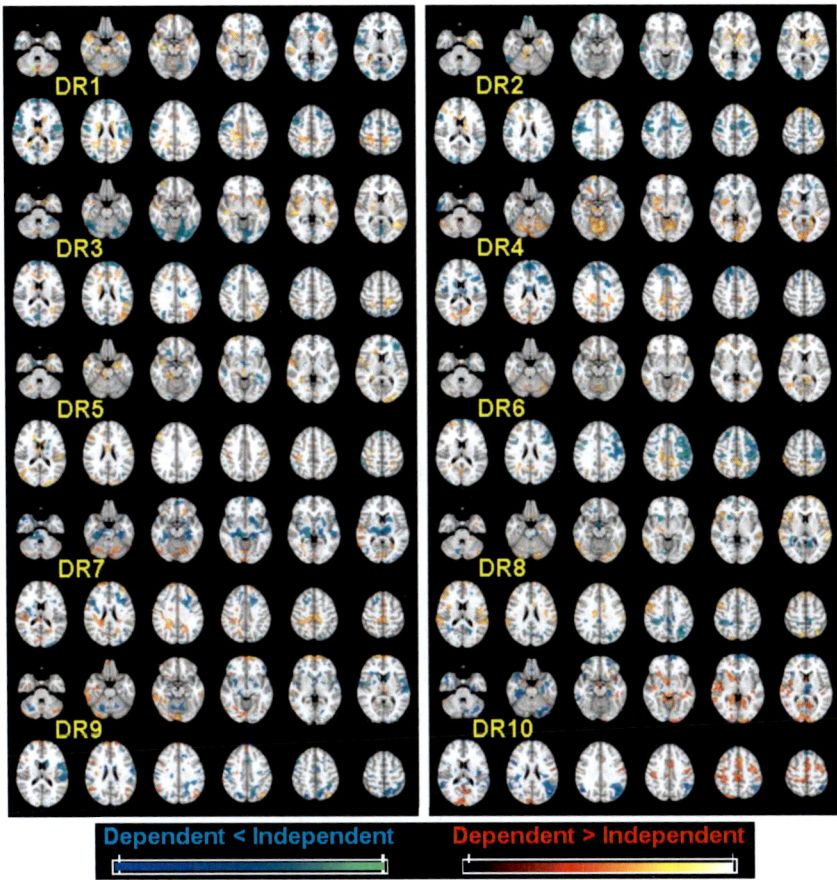

Figure 5. ICA-based DR with fMRI data found functional connectivity deficits in the regions related to language (frontal opercularis) function, motor/sensory, visual/frontal areas as well as salience network, substantia nigra, subcortical caudate thalamus and hypothalamus (DR components 1-10; blue: dependent group < independent group and red: dependent > independent group) in dependent compared to independent groups with P<0.01.

ICA-based DR algorithm detected intra- and inter- network connectivity deficits in the regions related to language (frontal opercularis) and communication function, motor/sensory, visual/frontal areas as well as salience network, frontoparietal network, substantia nigra, subcortical caudate, thalamus and hypothalamus in the dependent group compared to independent living participants (Figure5 for DR components 1-10 & Figure 6 for DR components 11-20). Typical compensated and rerouted regions of cerebellum, lingual and calcarine, supplementary motor area and dorsolateral prefrontal cortex presented higher functional connectivity (Figures 5, 6) in dependent compared to independent groups.

Statistical differences of tract-based diffusivity evaluation including radial diffusivity (RD), axial diffusivity (AD) and mean diffusivity (MD) between two participant groups are displayed in Figure 7. Higher RD, AD and MD values were found in dependent participants compared to independent group. Our results indicated possible demyelination in dependent living compared to independent participants (P = 0.02-0.04), shown as higher radial space quantified with RD in the corticospinal tract (motor function and somatosensory integration), cingulum (emotion, memory and various cognitive function), inferior fronto-occipital fasciculus (memory, language and executive function) as well as uncinate fasciculus (learning and memory, disinhibition behavior) in these patients. Moreover, axonal degeneration reflected with increased AD in the anterior thalamic radiation (prefrontal, premotor, motor and sensory projections), cortical spinal tract, inferior-occipital fasciculus and uncinate fasciculus were also present (P = 0.008-0.048). And finally the MD confirmed increased values (less white matter integrity) in these regions such as cingulum and the other three regions with both higher AD and RD (P = 0.01-0.04). All the tracts with increased diffusivity values were on the right side (R).

Cross-sectional and longitudinal DTI diffusivity differences at 1st initial visit between two group; as well as alterations between 1st and 2nd visits in each sub-group were demonstrated in Figure 8. Similar to the 2nd visit results as in Figure 7, diffusivity changes including higher RD, AD and MD in the right corticospinal tract and uncinate fasciculus were found in the dependent compared to independent groups at the initial visit (P < 0.05). Slightly decrease of AD in the right superior longitudinal fasciculus (SLF) temporal part was found in the dependent group (P = 0.04), possibly undergo Wallerian degeneration. Longitudinally, higher AD in the right corticospinal tract and left cingulum were also identified at 2nd visit compared to initial visit (P < 0.05) in the independent group that might be related to the aging effect and possible disease progression over time.

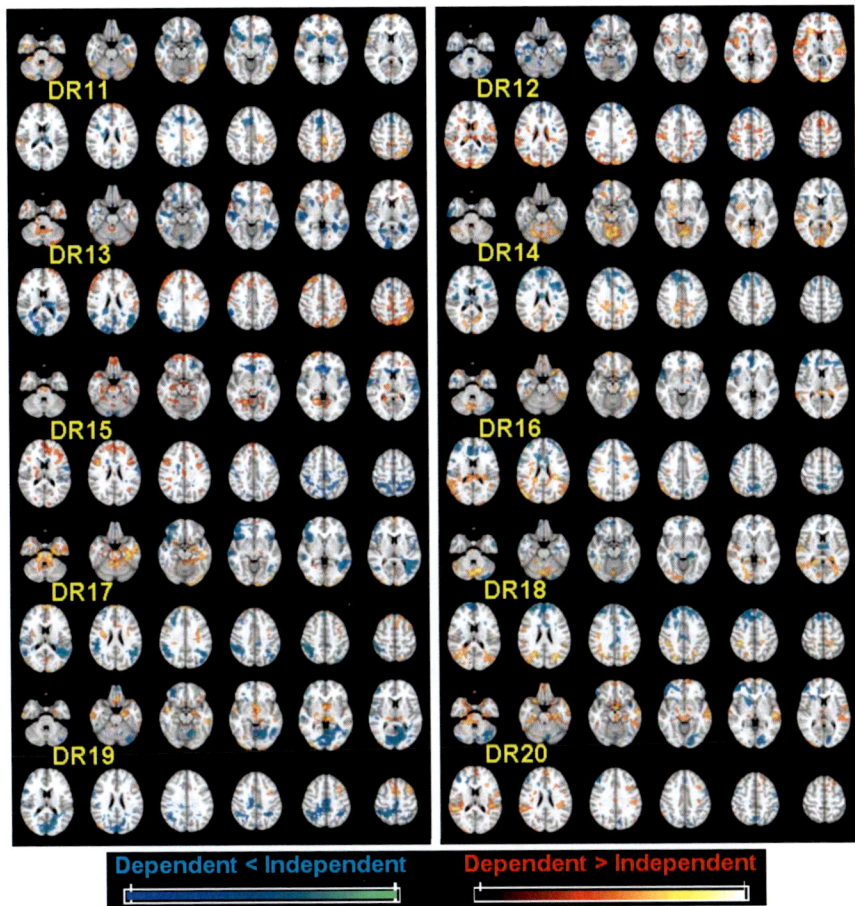

Figure 6. ICA-based DR results with fMRI data (DR components 11-20; blue: dependent < independent and red: dependent > independent) with P<0.01.

No other significant quantitative tract-based FA differences were found longitudinally in either of the two groups, neither as any cross-sectional difference between two groups at initial visit for the 20 tracts (P > 0.05). Whole brain voxel wise comparison using TBSS algorithm revealed no significant differences between two groups of diffusivity images including AD, RD and MD either. Summary of statistically significant tract-based diffusivity changes at both 1st and 2nd visits as well as longitudinal comparison between dependent and independent groups with P < 0.05 are listed in Table 3.

Finally, significantly higher global mean values of fALFF (a marker for neural activity) were found in the slow-wave sub-band S4 (0.027-0.073 Hz, P = 0.041) and conventional fALFF at low-frequency band (0.01-0.08 Hz, P = 0.007) in dependent compared to independent groups (Figure 9). Systematic analysis of RS-fMRI data based on small-worldness and network integration demonstrated higher local efficiency but lower global efficiency in dependent group compared to independent participants, and the resulted small-worldness factor was relatively lower in dependent group as well (Figure 10).

Table 3. Summary of significant DTI diffusivity changes (RD, AD and MD) between dependent and independent groups at 1st and 2nd visits as well as longitudinal comparisons in each group with P < 0.05

Tract of interest for quantification	RD (demyelination)	AD (axonal degeneration)	MD (overall integrity)
Comparison at 2nd visit (Figure 7)			
R Corticospinal tract (CST)	↑	↑	↑
R Cingulum	↑		↑
R Inferior fronto-occipital fasciculus	↑	↑	↑
R Uncinate fasciculus	↑	↑	↑
R Anterior thalamic radiation		↑	
Comparison at 1st visit (Figure 8)			
R Corticospinal tract (CST)	↑	↑	↑
R Uncinate fasciculus	↑	↑	↑
R Superior longitudinal fasciculus (TP)		↓ (Wallerian)	
Longitudinal comparison between 2nd and 1st visits (Figure 8; found only in independent group)			
R Corticospinal tract (CST)		↑	
L Cingulum		↑	

* R = right; L = left; TP = temporal part; ↑ denotes higher diffusivity in dependent compared to independent groups or 2nd > 1st visits for independent group; while ↓ for lower values at P < 0.05.

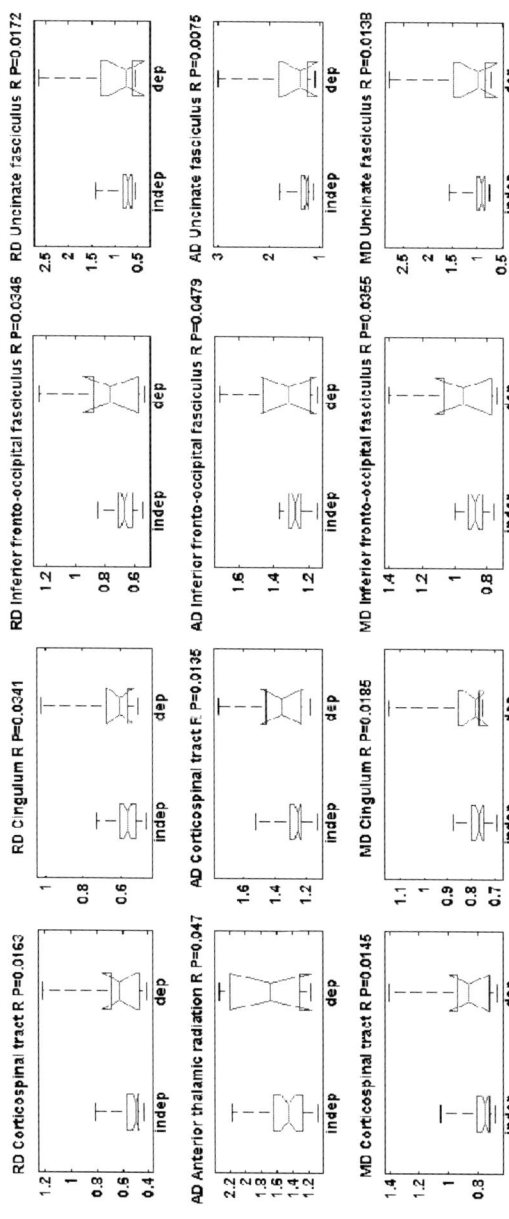

Figure 7. Statistical differences between two participant groups of diffusivity including radial diffusivity (RD), axial diffusivity (AD) and mean diffusivity (MD) were demonstrated. Higher RD, AD and MD were found in dependent participants compared to independent group. Our results indicated possible demyelination (1st row, higher radial space measured with RD) in the corticospinal tract (motor function), cingulum (emotion, memory, and various cognitive function), inferior fronto-occipital fasciculus (memory, language and executive function) as well as uncinate fasciculus (learning and memory, possible disinhibition behavior) in dependent living compared to independent groups (P = 0.02-0.04). Axonal degeneration (2nd row) with increased AD in the anterior thalamic radiation (prefrontal, premotor, motor and sensory projections), and other three tracts that had higher RD as well including cortical spinal tract, inferior-occipital fasciculus and uncinate fasciculus were also present (P = 0.008-0.048). And finally, the mean diffusivity (MD, 3rd row) confirmed increased values (less white matter integrity) in these tracts such as cingulum and the other three fiber bundles showing both higher AD and RD as in 1st and 2d panel (P = 0.01-0.04). All the tracts with increased diffusivity values were on the right side (R).

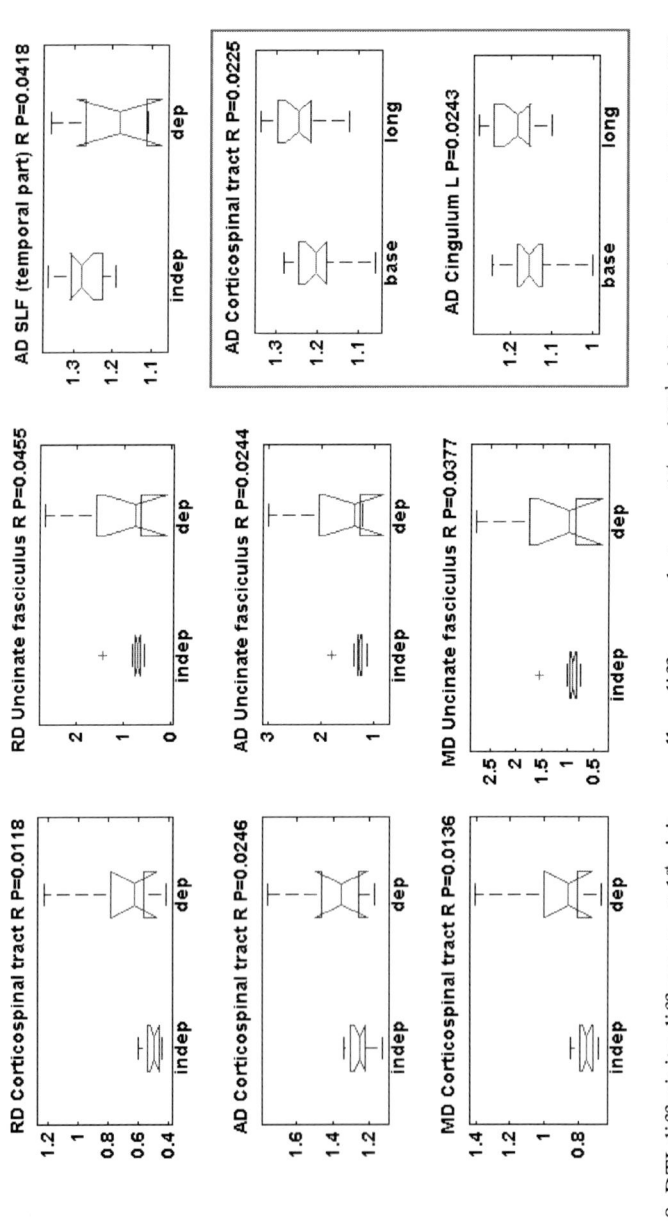

Figure 8. DTI diffusivity differences at 1st visit; as well as differences between 1st and 2nd visits in red rectangle. No FA differences were identified longitudinally visit (long) or at baseline (base). In the initial visit, similar diffusivity changes as to 2nd visit between independent (indep.) and dependent (dep.) groups were identified including higher RD, AD and MD in the dependent group in the right cortical spinal and uncinate fasciculus tracts (P < 0.05). Slightly decrease of AD in the right superior longitudinal fasciculus (SLF), temporal part was found in the dependent compared to independent groups (P = 0.04), possibly undergo Wallerian degeneration. Longitudinally, in the independent group, higher AD of the right corticospinal tract and left cingulum were identified at 2nd visit compared to initial visit (P < 0.05; red rectangle box), possibly due to the aging effect and disease progression over time.

Table 4. Summary of significant MRI/PET alterations including VBM, VMHC, DR-ICA and DTI MRI metrics together with PET molecular tracers for dopamine transporter (DAT) and striatal binding ratio (SBR) as well as VMAT2 densities and amyloid/FDG uptake in patients of PD, FTD and VaD compared to controls including sub-types and different conditions.

Metric	VBM GM Density (GMD)	VMHC (Interhemispheric Functional Conductivity)	ICA-DR (Intra- and Inter- Network Functional Connectivity)	More MRI Quantifications (DTI, fALFF SMW) and PET Molecular Tracers
PD (GPD & PM)	* Lower GMD (atrophy) in inferior and middle temporal cortex, medial-orbito frontal cortex, dorsolateral prefrontal cortex motor and supplementary motor cortices in PD vs. NC * Higher in small clusters in cerebellum, insular, posterior putamen and basal ganglia * Lower fALFF in PD (S4 and conventional) vs. GPD	* Lower in the basal ganglia including the swallow tail signs in the substantia nigra, red nucleus, hypothalamus, thalamus, ventral striatum, caudate, lingual gyrus, postcentral gyrus, rectus and temporal cortex. * Higher in middle and superio-frontal, middle cingulate, fusiform, motor and supplementary motor cortices, superior parietal and occipital cortices * GPD similar to PD (less lower but more positive regions in GPD) and PM (lower VMHC in majority of brain areas)	* Lower network connectivity in the DMN regions and subcortical caudate and thalamus regions, basal ganglia and temporal/orbitofrontal regions, motor as well as supplementary motor cortex and superior/medial frontal regions. * Higher in inter-frontal and dorsolateral prefrontal network motor/ supplementary cortices, temporal and occipital regions, basal ganglia related motor region. * GPD similar to PD; PM presented stronger hypo- and hyper- network connectivity in GPD/PD vs. NC	* Lower FA in right substantia nigra (middle portion) in PD vs. NC * Higher local efficiency with slightly lower relative global efficiency in PD compared to NC * Lower (~50%) dopamine SBR and DAT levels in PD vs. NC in striatal caudate and putamen regions. * Lower VMAT2 in PD/GPD vs. NC in caudate, mesial temporal cortex, left frontal such as orbitofrontal and occipital cortices

Table 4. (Continued)

Metric	VBM GM Density (GMD)	VMHC (Interhemispheric Functional Conductivity)	ICA-DR (Intra- and Inter- Network Functional Connectivity)	More MRI Quantifications (DTI, fALFF SMW) and PET Molecular Tracers
FTD including opening vs. closing eyes and longitudinal comparisons	* Atrophy in orbitofrontal cortex, scattered temporal regions, medial prefrontal, striatum including putamen and caudate, insular, motor, dorsolateral attentional regions such as prefrontal cortex, and superior parietal cortex * Lower FA in the genu of corpus callosum, both limbs of the internal capsule, small clusters in cerebral peduncle and sagittal striatum	* Lower in temporal, visual, orbitofrontal and parietal cortices; higher in cerebellum, dorsolateral attention network, salience network including insular, superior frontal and parietal regions in FTD * Lower in large areas in the subcortical caudate, thalamus, hypothalamus, insular, parietal, visual, frontal motor/premotor and temporal regions including amygdala at opening vs. closing eyes relaxing condition * Lower in inferior parietal, temporal, insular, superior frontal, cuneus and calcarine areas longitudinally	* Lower in FTD vs. NC in cerebellum, temporal and occipital regions, insular, superior frontal and posterior DMN regions together with frontoparietal network * Higher in thalamus and dorsolateral prefrontal cortex as well as some motor and supplementary motor regions * Higher inter-DMN and DAN modulation, motor/premotor network vs. Lower temporal, visual, insular, fronto-parietal network and striato-thalamo-cortical regions for opening vs. closing eyes * Lower in temporal cortex (hippocampus), orbito and medial prefrontal cortices longitudinally, higher in DAN & cerebellum	* Higher amyloid burden in temporal and frontal regions in bvFTD vs. NC * FDG hypometabolism in orbitofrontal and medial prefrontal cortices, multiple temporal regions including amygdala and hippocampus, thalamus, anterior and middle cingulate, insular, fronto-parietal and dorsal attentional networks (DAN) * Lower local but higher global efficiency in FTD * Lower local and global at opening vs. closing eyes situation in FTD
VaD (Dependent vs. Independent group)	* Atrophy in orbitofrontal, temporal, medial frontal, superior frontal gyrus and middle occipital cortices; * Higher in subcortical thalamus, middle cingulate, postcentral sensory, motor and pons areas	* Monotonically lower in large regions of inferior parietal, dorsolateral prefrontal and orbital frontal such as the triangularis and opercularis regions, frontal pole, visual cortex, basal ganglia, thalamus, cerebellum, anterior temporal cortex and motor areas in dependent compared to independent groups	* Lower in, opercularis, visual/frontal, motor/sensory, salience network, frontoparietal network, substantia nigra, subcortical caudate, thalamus and hypothalamus * Higher in cerebellum supplementary motor area, lingual and calcarine and dorsolateral prefrontal cortex in dependent compared to independent groups	* Higher local efficiency but lower global efficiency in dependent compared to independent groups * Higher fALFF (S4 sub-band and conventional) * Higher AD/RD in corticospinal tract, cingulum, inferior fronto-occipital & uncinate fasciculus

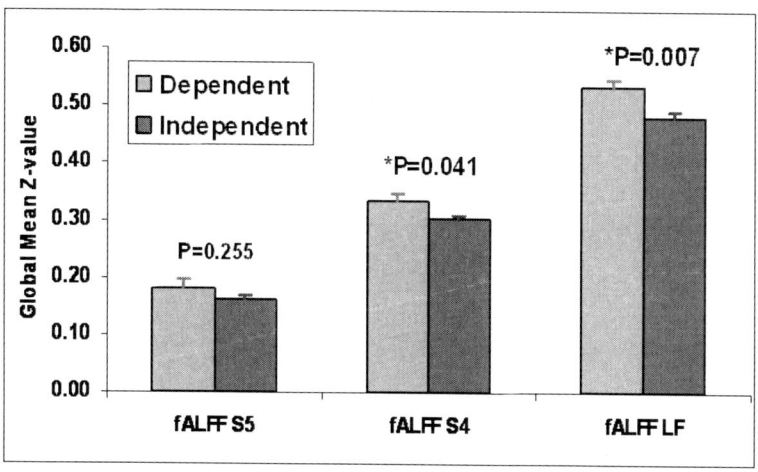

Figure 9. fALFF differences between two groups at low frequency slow-waves sub-band of S5 (0.01-0.027 Hz) and S4 (0.027-0.073 Hz), as well as conventional low frequency (LF) of 0.01-0.08Hz. Significantly higher global mean values of fALFF were found in the slow-wave band S4 (P = 0.041) and conventional LF fALFF (P = 0.007) in dependent compared to independent groups.

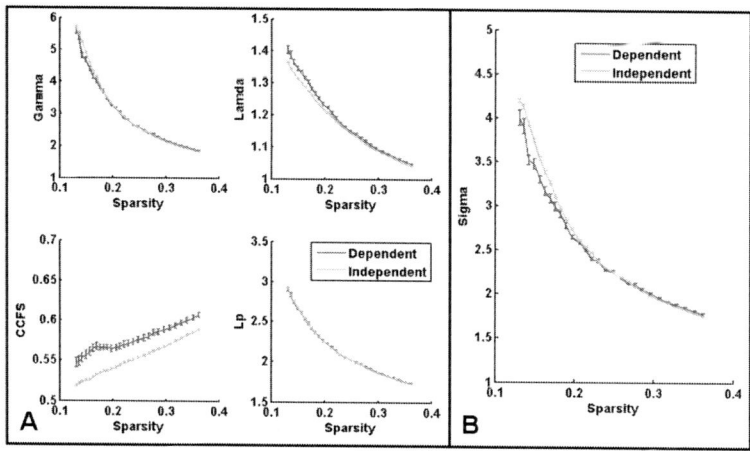

Figure 10. A: Small-worldness based systematic analysis of RS-fMRI data demonstrated higher absolute local efficiency (CCFS, red dark line) in dependent group compared to independent participants (blue light line). On the other hand, lower relative global efficiencies (Lamda) in dependent group with longer relative shortest path length. Gamma and Lp values were quite close in two groups. B: The scaled small-worldness factor (Sigma) was lower in dependent compared to independent groups, especially at low sparsity level (0.12-0.2 range).

4. Discussion

4.1. Summary of Results

Lower FA in the corpus callosum and abnormal values in scattered tracts such as the superior longitudinal fasciculus, corticospinal tract, uncinate fasciculus and cingulum were found in dependent compared to independent groups. Moreover, atrophy in the orbitofrontal, temporal, medial frontal and middle occipital cortices were present in the dependent group, accompanied with higher gray matter density in subcortical and basal ganglia as well as the middle cingulum regions. Similar but larger spatial distributions of brain regions of inferior parietal, dorsolateral prefrontal and orbital frontal cortices, basal ganglia including substantia nigra, amygdala, hypothalamus, thalamus, cerebellum, anterior temporal cortex, posterior cingulate, motor area and visual cortex exhibited monotonically and significantly lower VMHC values in the dependent group, reflecting discoordination, demyelination and slowness of information processing speed. ICA-DR identified functional connectivity deficits in the regions related to language function (frontal opercularis), motor/sensory, visual/frontal areas as well as salience network, substantia nigra, subcortical caudate, thalamus and hypothalamus in the dependent group as well. On the other hand, typical regions of cerebellum, supplementary motor area, visual and dorsal attentional networks presented higher functional connectivity in dependent compared to independent group for neuroprotection and network rerouting. Increased global mean neuronal activity with higher fALFF in the slow-wave sub-band S4 and conventional low frequency band (0.01-0.08Hz) in dependent group compared to independent group indicated more neuronal resource utilization for possible compensation and disinhibition or over-activity in local regions in patients. This had been further validated in dependent group with less efficiency of systematic integration (i.e., lower global but higher local efficiency) based on small-worldness analysis.

Furthermore, higher RD and MD in the corticospinal tract, cingulum, inferior fronto-occipital fasciculus as well as uncinate fasciculus were found in the dependent group compared to independent group, indicating possible demyelination causing movement disorder, disinhibition behavior, emotion, learning and memory and high-level cognitive impairments together with executive function and attention deficits in these patients. Higher AD in additional anterior thalamic radiation tract (not cingulum) was found relating to prefrontal, premotor, motor and sensory functionality, indicating axonal degeneration in addition to the demyelination in these areas. All the alterations were on the right side laterally, consistent with previous imaging findings in VaD patients [14, 16]. Higher RD, AD and MD in the right corticospinal and uncinate fasciculus tracts were also found in the dependent group at initial visit; confirming the long-term white matter degeneration in the primary tracts for basic brain function such as motor control, inhibition, learning and memory. The AD of right superior longitudinal fasciculus (temporal part) was lower in the dependent group (with slightly lower FA in TBSS results), indicating retrograde Wallerian degeneration in the memory-connected fiber initially. Longitudinally, higher AD in the right corticospinal tract (similar to the findings of both visits in dependent group) and left cingulum were identified in the independent group, reflecting possible disease progression and aging effects [26].

4.2. Comparison with Previous Findings – MRI/fMRI/DTI/PET Multimodal Results

In frail elderly persons, DTI alterations were found in large areas of white matter and were strongly associated with WMH in comparison to nonfrail subgroup [27]. Similarly, DTI and age-related white matter changes were convergent and presented widespread WM changes in participants with early cerebral microangiopathy; together with gray matter atrophy in frontal areas [28]. Lower WM integrity with reduced FA values and high mean diffusivity in genu and splenium of the corpus callosum were observed in subcortical vascular dementia of Binswanger type (SVaD-BT) patients [29]. In stroke patients, consistent distribution pattern of leukoaraiosis was strongly associated with risk of incident stroke and dementia, possibly resulted from the vulnerability to WM injury across various vascular diseases [30]. It had been found that WMH was connected with episodic memory, and reflecting ischemic pathology in chronic obstructive pulmonary disease [31]. And furthermore, by including trauma lesion location information, significant correlations existed between WM injury and cognitive tests [32]. WMH accumulation over time in SVD, especially in the frontal areas, might be due to the lesions in the centrum semiovale and striatum; and incorporating hippocampal gray matter density could achieve classification accuracy of 73% [33].

Structurally, gray matter (GM) atrophy was distributed in both cortical regions and subcortical areas in VaD [34]. For instance, frontal and occipital atrophies including frontal pole, precentral gyrus and medial prefrontal cortex (MFPC) as well as the lingual gyrus were found in SVaD-BT patients, followed by temporal atrophy such as in the fusiform and middle temporal gyrus [29]. Another study also confirmed the widespread GM atrophy in frontal cortex such as MPFC and inferior temporal cortex in SVaD, as well as several subcortical regions such as thalamus and caudate [35]. Functionally, decreased fMRI activation in prefrontal cortex in response to the Stroop task compared to controls was observed in SVaD [36]. Lower functional connectivities were also found in SVaD, including between the thalamus and the orbitofrontal cortex as well as between MPFC and supplementary motor area, accompanied by the higher inferior frontal connectivity for possible compensatory [34]. Lower intra- default mode network (DMN) hippocampal functional connectivity but higher intra- central executive-function network (CEN) connections were observed in VaD patients compared to controls [37].

Regarding VMHC and fALFF findings, disrupted VMHC between the bilateral lingual gyrus, putamen and precentral gyrus were found in SVaD patients [38]. For fALFF, lower values in the anterior DMN but higher in the posterior portion in SVaD were found, and insular fALFF value was associated with cognitive and memory scores [35, 39, 40]. And finally, the small-worldness network analysis identified disrupted global topological organization of the functional brain networks in SVaD compared to controls, with lower global and local efficiencies measured by reduced clustering coefficients and increased characteristic path lengths relative to normal subjects [41]. Revealing brain network changes involving key cortical such as prefrontal cortex and subcortical regions including basal ganglia and cerebellum might help understand disease mechanism and discover better rehabilitative strategies for dependent individuals [42].

4.3. Future Works

Due to the limited number of participants in dependent group, the results presented in this work are still preliminary. Expanding to large data cohort and connecting with the clinical data will be some future works. Integrating white matter lesion quantification could improve disease diagnosis, and applying the automatic lesion segmentation algorithm as shown by a recent work of 0.94 accuracy will be considered [43]. Furthermore, utilization of relatively new imaging techniques such as combination of MRI and PET molecular imaging results with simultaneous PET/MRI, and quantitative blood flow analysis from arterial spin labeling technique might help better elucidate the underlying pathophysiological process of diseases including stroke, VaD and dependence/disability [44-46].

In conclusion, we had reported multiparametric imaging abnormalities in the dependent group compared to independent participants in the VaD data cohort, including lower FA, lower VMHC, brain atrophy and functional connectivity deficits, higher neural activity coherence as well as lower neuronal source utilization efficiency in these patients. Furthermore, higher diffusivity values of AD, RD and MD in dependent compared to independent groups at initial and follow-up visits in certain brain tracts including cingulum, corticospinal tract and uncinate fasciculus for memory, movement and inhibition connectivity were identified, suggesting white matter integrity damage such as demyelination, axonal and Wallerian degeneration in the dependent group. Our results were consistent with previously reported findings in general VaD, and provided systematic, comprehensive and quantitative neuropathological and neurophysiological clues to the disease severity.

And more specifically, our combined MRI/PET results had presented unique region/pattern and brain circuit feature for distinguishing each type of neurodegenerative disease. The summary of the main MRI/PET findings in three types of general neurodegenerative diseases including VaD in this chapter and PD in Chapters 1 and 2 together with FTD in Chapter 3, is listed in Table 4. For instance, motor, frontal and basal ganglia system breakdown in PD, frontal and temporal regional deficits including atrophy, hypometabolism and network hypoconnectivity as well as dis-coordination in FTD; and finally frontal and visual brain circuits deterioration together with white matter injury in VaD dependent group were illustrated. The relatively new VMHC for myelin-related conductivity measure and ICA-DR intra-/inter- network remapping methods in addition to the numerous quantifications (neuronal activity, systematic efficiency, tract-based diffusivity, glucose/amyloid and dopamine levels) had proved to be valid diagnosis tool for general clinical disease applications.

REFERENCES

[1] Prosser AMJ, Spreadbury JH, Tossici-Bolt L, Kipps CM. Imaging Care Requirements: Use of Functional Neuroimaging to Predict Dementia Caregiver Burden. *Dement Geriatr Cogn Dis Extra.* 2018 Apr 26;8(1):180-189. doi: 10.1159/000486479. PMID: 29805384; PMCID: PMC5968276.

[2] Heiss WD, Kidwell CS. Imaging for prediction of functional outcome and assessment of recovery in ischemic stroke. *Stroke.* 2014 Apr;45(4):1195-201. doi: 10.1161/STROKEAHA.113.003611. Epub 2014 Mar 4. PMID: 24595589; PMCID: PMC3981064.

[3] Niewada M, Członkowska A. Prevention of ischemic stroke in clinical practice: a role of internists and general practitioners. *Pol Arch Med Wewn.* 2014;124(10):540-8. doi: 10.20452/pamw.2464. PMID: 25369511.

[4] Wardlaw JM, Smith C, Dichgans M. Mechanisms of sporadic cerebral small vessel disease: insights from neuroimaging. *Lancet Neurol.* 2013 May; 12(5):483-97. doi: 10.1016/S1474-4422(13)70060-7. Erratum in: *Lancet Neurol.* 2013 Jun;12(6):532. PMID: 23602162; PMCID: PMC3836247.

[5] Sachdev P, Kalaria R, O'Brien J, Skoog I, Alladi S, Black SE, Blacker D, Blazer DG, Chen C, Chui H, Ganguli M, Jellinger K, Jeste DV, Pasquier F, Paulsen J, Prins N, Rockwood K, Roman G, Scheltens P; Internationlal Society for Vascular Behavioral and Cognitive Disorders. Diagnostic criteria for vascular cognitive disorders: a VASCOG statement. *Alzheimer Dis Assoc Disord.* 2014 Jul-Sep;28(3):206-18. doi: 10.1097/WAD.0000000000000034. PMID: 24632990; PMCID: PMC4139434.

[6] Gorelick PB, Counts SE, Nyenhuis D. Vascular cognitive impairment and dementia. *Biochim Biophys Acta.* 2016 May;1862 (5):860-8. doi: 10.1016/j.bbadis.2015.12.015. Epub 2015 Dec 15. PMID: 26704177; PMCID: PMC5232167.

[7] Shabir O, Berwick J, Francis SE. Neurovascular dysfunction in vascular dementia, Alzheimer's and atherosclerosis. *BMC Neurosci.* 2018 Oct 17;19(1):62. doi: 10.1186/s12868-018-0465-5. PMID: 30333009; PMCID: PMC6192291.

[8] Kalaria RN. Neuropathological diagnosis of vascular cognitive impairment and vascular dementia with implications for Alzheimer's disease. *Acta Neuropathol.* 2016 May;131(5):659-85. doi: 10.1007/s00401-016-1571-z. Epub 2016 Apr 9. PMID: 27062261; PMCID: PMC4835512.

[9] Sargurupremraj M, Suzuki H, Jian X, Sarnowski C, Evans TE, Bis JC, Eiriksdottir G, Sakaue S, Terzikhan N, Habes M, Zhao W, Armstrong NJ, Hofer E, Yanek LR, Hagenaars SP, Kumar RB, van den Akker EB, McWhirter RE, Trompet S, Mishra A, Saba Y, Satizabal CL, Beaudet G, Petit L, Tsuchida A, Zago L, Schilling S, Sigurdsson S, Gottesman RF, Lewis CE, Aggarwal NT, Lopez OL, Smith JA, Valdés Hernández MC, van der Grond J, Wright MJ, Knol MJ, Dörr M, Thomson RJ, Bordes C, Le Grand Q, Duperron MG,

Smith AV, Knopman DS, Schreiner PJ, Evans DA, Rotter JI, Beiser AS, Maniega SM, Beekman M, Trollor J, Stott DJ, Vernooij MW, Wittfeld K, Niessen WJ, Soumaré A, Boerwinkle E, Sidney S, Turner ST, Davies G, Thalamuthu A, Völker U, van Buchem MA, Bryan RN, Dupuis J, Bastin ME, Ames D, Teumer A, Amouyel P, Kwok JB, Bülow R, Deary IJ, Schofield PR, Brodaty H, Jiang J, Tabara Y, Setoh K, Miyamoto S, Yoshida K, Nagata M, Kamatani Y, Matsuda F, Psaty BM, Bennett DA, De Jager PL, Mosley TH, Sachdev PS, Schmidt R, Warren HR, Evangelou E, Trégouët DA; International Network against Thrombosis (INVENT) Consortium; International Headache Genomics Consortium (IHGC), Ikram MA, Wen W, DeCarli C, Srikanth VK, Jukema JW, Slagboom EP, Kardia SLR, Okada Y, Mazoyer B, Wardlaw JM, Nyquist PA, Mather KA, Grabe HJ, Schmidt H, Van Duijn CM, Gudnason V, Longstreth WT Jr, Launer LJ, Lathrop M, Seshadri S, Tzourio C, Adams HH, Matthews PM, Fornage M, Debette S. Cerebral small vessel disease genomics and its implications across the lifespan. *Nat Commun.* 2020 Dec 8;11(1):6285. doi: 10.1038/s41467-020-19111-2. PMID: 33293549; PMCID: PMC7722866.

[10] Zhou Y, Yu F, Duong TQ; Alzheimer's Disease Neuroimaging Initiative. White matter lesion load is associated with resting state functional MRI activity and amyloid PET but not FDG in mild cognitive impairment and early Alzheimer's disease patients. *J Magn Reson Imaging.* 2015 Jan;41(1):102-9. doi: 10.1002/jmri.24550. Epub 2013 Dec 31. PMID: 24382798; PMCID: PMC4097981.

[11] Moreton FC, Cullen B, Delles C, Santosh C, Gonzalez RL, Dani K, Muir KW. Vasoreactivity in CADASIL: Comparison to structural MRI and neuropsychology. *J Cereb Blood Flow Metab.* 2018 Jun;38(6):1085-1095. doi: 10.1177/0271678X17710375. Epub 2017 May 24. PMID: 28537106; PMCID: PMC5998994.

[12] Zhou Y. *Neuroimaging in Multiple Sclerosis.* Nova Science Publishers. 2017.

[13] Lambert C, Zeestraten E, Williams O, Benjamin P, Lawrence AJ, Morris RG, Mackinnon AD, Barrick TR, Markus HS. Identifying

preclinical vascular dementia in symptomatic small vessel disease using MRI. *Neuroimage Clin.* 2018 Jun 20;19:925-938. doi: 10.1016/j.nicl.2018.06.023. PMID: 30003030; PMCID: PMC6039843.

[14] Migliaccio R, Tanguy D, Bouzigues A, Sezer I, Dubois B, Le Ber I, Batrancourt B, Godefroy V, Levy R. Cognitive and behavioural inhibition deficits in neurodegenerative dementias. *Cortex.* 2020 Oct;131:265-283. doi: 10.1016/j.cortex.2020.08.001. Epub 2020 Aug 10. PMID: 32919754; PMCID: PMC7416687.

[15] Hughes LE, Rittman T, Robbins TW, Rowe JB. Reorganization of cortical oscillatory dynamics underlying disinhibition in frontotemporal dementia. *Brain.* 2018 Aug 1;141(8):2486-2499. doi: 10.1093/brain/awy176. PMID: 29992242; PMCID: PMC6061789.

[16] Rosen HJ, Allison SC, Schauer GF, Gorno-Tempini ML, Weiner MW, Miller BL. Neuroanatomical correlates of behavioural disorders in dementia. *Brain.* 2005 Nov;128(Pt 11):2612-25. doi: 10.1093/brain/awh628. Epub 2005 Sep 29. PMID: 16195246; PMCID: PMC1820861.

[17] Hornberger M, Geng J, Hodges JR. Convergent grey and white matter evidence of orbitofrontal cortex changes related to disinhibition in behavioural variant frontotemporal dementia. *Brain.* 2011 Sep;134(Pt 9):2502-12. doi: 10.1093/brain/awr173. Epub 2011 Jul 23. PMID: 21785117.

[18] Heiss WD, Rosenberg GA, Thiel A, Berlot R, de Reuck J. Neuroimaging in vascular cognitive impairment: a state-of-the-art review. *BMC Med.* 2016 Nov 3;14(1):174. doi: 10.1186/s12916-016-0725-0. PMID: 27806705; PMCID: PMC5094143.

[19] Duering M, Finsterwalder S, Baykara E, Tuladhar AM, Gesierich B, Konieczny MJ, Malik R, Franzmeier N, Ewers M, Jouvent E, Biessels GJ, Schmidt R, de Leeuw FE, Pasternak O, Dichgans M. Free water determines diffusion alterations and clinical status in cerebral small vessel disease. *Alzheimers Dement.* 2018 Jun;14(6): 764-774. doi: 10.1016/j.jalz.2017.12.007. Epub 2018 Feb 16. PMID: 29406155; PMCID: PMC5994358.

[20] Wong SM, Zhang CE, van Bussel FC, Staals J, Jeukens CR, Hofman PA, van Oostenbrugge RJ, Backes WH, Jansen JF. Simultaneous investigation of microvasculature and parenchyma in cerebral small vessel disease using intravoxel incoherent motion imaging. *Neuroimage Clin.* 2017 Jan 17;14:216-221. doi: 10.1016/j.nicl. 2017.01.017. PMID: 28180080; PMCID: PMC5288390.

[21] Brookes RL, Herbert V, Lawrence AJ, Morris RG, Markus HS. Depression in small-vessel disease relates to white matter ultrastructural damage, not disability. *Neurology.* 2014 Oct 14;83(16):1417-23. doi: 10.1212/WNL.0000000000000882. Epub 2014 Sep 17. PMID: 25230999; PMCID: PMC4206159.

[22] Lamar M, Zhou XJ, Charlton RA, Dean D, Little D, Deoni SC. In vivo quantification of white matter microstructure for use in aging: a focus on two emerging techniques. *Am J Geriatr Psychiatry.* 2014 Feb;22(2):111-21. doi: 10.1016/j.jagp.2013.08.001. Epub 2013 Sep 27. PMID: 24080382; PMCID: PMC3947219.

[23] Ji F, Pasternak O, Liu S, Loke YM, Choo BL, Hilal S, Xu X, Ikram MK, Venketasubramanian N, Chen CL, Zhou J. Distinct white matter microstructural abnormalities and extracellular water increases relate to cognitive impairment in Alzheimer's disease with and without cerebrovascular disease. *Alzheimers Res Ther.* 2017 Aug 17;9(1):63. doi: 10.1186/s13195-017-0292-4. PMID: 28818116; PMCID: PMC5561637.

[24] Du J, Wang Y, Zhi N, Geng J, Cao W, Yu L, Mi J, Zhou Y, Xu Q, Wen W, Sachdev P. Structural brain network measures are superior to vascular burden scores in predicting early cognitive impairment in post stroke patients with small vessel disease. *Neuroimage Clin.* 2019;22:101712. doi: 10.1016/j.nicl.2019.101712. Epub 2019 Feb 5. PMID: 30772684; PMCID: PMC6378318.

[25] Zhou Y. *Functional Neuroimaging with Multiple Modalities: Principle, Device and Applicaitons*. Nova Science Publishers. 2016.

[26] Zhou Y. *Function and Metabolism at Aging: Longitudinal Neuroimaging Evaluations*. Nova Science Publishers. 2019.

[27] Avila-Funes JA, Pelletier A, Meillon C, Catheline G, Periot O, Trevin O-Frenk I, Gonzalez-Colaço M, Dartigues JF, Pérès K, Allard M, Dilharreguy B, Amieva H. Vascular Cerebral Damage in Frail Older Adults: The AMImage Study. *J Gerontol A Biol Sci Med Sci.* 2017 Jul 1;72(7):971-977. doi: 10.1093/gerona/glw347. PMID: 28329104.

[28] Quinque EM, Arélin K, Dukart J, Roggenhofer E, Streitbuerger DP, Villringer A, Frisch S, Mueller K, Schroeter ML. Identifying the neural correlates of executive functions in early cerebral microangiopathy: a combined VBM and DTI study. *J Cereb Blood Flow Metab.* 2012 Oct;32(10):1869-78. doi: 10.1038/jcbfm.2012.96. Epub 2012 Jul 11. PMID: 22781332; PMCID: PMC3463884.

[29] Jung WB, Mun CW, Kim YH, Park JM, Lee BD, Lee YM, Moon E, Jeong HJ, Chung YI. Cortical atrophy, reduced integrity of white matter and cognitive impairment in subcortical vascular dementia of Binswanger type. *Psychiatry Clin Neurosci.* 2014 Dec;68(12):821-832. doi: 10.1111/pcn.12196. Epub 2014 Aug 6. PMID: 24773562.

[30] Smith EE. Leukoaraiosis and stroke. *Stroke.* 2010 Oct;41(10 Suppl):S139-43. doi: 10.1161/STROKEAHA.110.596056. PMID: 20876490; PMCID: PMC2958335.

[31] Spilling CA, Jones PW, Dodd JW, Barrick TR. White matter lesions characterise brain involvement in moderate to severe chronic obstructive pulmonary disease, but cerebral atrophy does not. *BMC Pulm Med.* 2017 Jun 19;17(1):92. doi: 10.1186/s12890-017-0435-1. PMID: 28629404; PMCID: PMC5474872.

[32] Kuceyeski A, Maruta J, Niogi SN, Ghajar J, Raj A. The generation and validation of white matter connectivity importance maps. *Neuroimage.* 2011 Sep 1;58(1):109-21. doi: 10.1016/j.neuroimage.2011.05.087. Epub 2011 Jun 29. PMID: 21722739; PMCID: PMC3144270.

[33] Lambert C, Zeestraten E, Williams O, Benjamin P, Lawrence AJ, Morris RG, Mackinnon AD, Barrick TR, Markus HS. Identifying preclinical vascular dementia in symptomatic small vessel disease using MRI. *Neuroimage Clin.* 2018 Jun 20;19:925-938. doi:

10.1016/j.nicl.2018.06.023. PMID: 30003030; PMCID: PMC6039843.

[34] Zhou X, Hu X, Zhang C, Wang H, Zhu X, Xu L, Sun Z, Yu Y. Aberrant Functional Connectivity and Structural Atrophy in Subcortical Vascular Cognitive Impairment: Relationship with Cognitive Impairments. *Front Aging Neurosci.* 2016 Feb 2;8:14. doi: 10.3389/fnagi.2016.00014. PMID: 26869922; PMCID: PMC4736471.

[35] Yi L, Wang J, Jia L, Zhao Z, Lu J, Li K, Jia J, He Y, Jiang C, Han Y. Structural and functional changes in subcortical vascular mild cognitive impairment: a combined voxel-based morphometry and resting-state fMRI study. *PLoS One.* 2012;7(9):e44758. doi: 10.1371/journal.pone.0044758. Epub 2012 Sep 19. PMID: 23028606; PMCID: PMC3446994.

[36] Li C, Zheng J, Wang J. An fMRI study of prefrontal cortical function in subcortical ischemic vascular cognitive impairment. *Am J Alzheimers Dis Other Demen.* 2012 Nov;27(7):490-5. doi: 10.1177/1533317512455841. Epub 2012 Aug 7. PMID: 22871909.

[37] Vipin A, Loke YM, Liu S, Hilal S, Shim HY, Xu X, Tan BY, Venketasubramanian N, Chen CL, Zhou J. Cerebrovascular disease influences functional and structural network connectivity in patients with amnestic mild cognitive impairment and Alzheimer's disease. *Alzheimers Res Ther.* 2018 Aug 18;10(1):82. doi: 10.1186/s13195-018-0413-8. PMID: 30121086; PMCID: PMC6098837.

[38] Ding W, Cao W, Wang Y, Sun Y, Chen X, Zhou Y, Xu Q, Xu J. Altered Functional Connectivity in Patients with Subcortical Vascular Cognitive Impairment--A Resting-State Functional Magnetic Resonance Imaging Study. *PLoS One.* 2015 Sep 16;10(9):e0138180. doi: 10.1371/journal.pone.0138180. PMID: 26376180; PMCID: PMC4573963.

[39] Liu C, Li C, Yin X, Yang J, Zhou D, Gui L, Wang J. Abnormal intrinsic brain activity patterns in patients with subcortical ischemic vascular dementia. *PLoS One.* 2014 Feb 3;9(2):e87880. doi: 10.1371/journal.pone.0087880. PMID: 24498389; PMCID: PMC3912127.

[40] Su J, Wang M, Ban S, Wang L, Cheng X, Hua F, Tang Y, Zhou H, Zhai Y, Du X, Liu J. Relationship between changes in resting-state spontaneous brain activity and cognitive impairment in patients with CADASIL. *J Headache Pain.* 2019 Apr 17;20(1):36. doi: 10.1186/s10194-019-0982-3. PMID: 30995925; PMCID: PMC6734224.

[41] Yu Y, Zhou X, Wang H, Hu X, Zhu X, Xu L, Zhang C, Sun Z. Small-World Brain Network and Dynamic Functional Distribution in Patients with Subcortical Vascular Cognitive Impairment. *PLoS One.* 2015 Jul 1;10(7):e0131893. doi: 10.1371/journal.pone.0131893. PMID: 26132397; PMCID: PMC4489389.

[42] Allali G, Blumen HM, Devanne H, Pirondini E, Delval A, Van De Ville D. Brain imaging of locomotion in neurological conditions. *Neurophysiol Clin.* 2018 Dec;48(6):337-359. doi: 10.1016/j.neucli.2018.10.004. Epub 2018 Oct 25. PMID: 30487063; PMCID: PMC6563601.

[43] Chen L, Bentley P, Rueckert D. Fully automatic acute ischemic lesion segmentation in DWI using convolutional neural networks. Neuroimage Clin. 2017 Jun 13;15:633-643. doi: 10.1016/j.nicl.2017.06.016. PMID: 28664034; PMCID: PMC5480013.

[44] Anazodo UC, Finger E, Kwan BYM, Pavlosky W, Warrington JC, Günther M, Prato FS, Thiessen JD, St Lawrence KS. Using simultaneous PET/MRI to compare the accuracy of diagnosing frontotemporal dementia by arterial spin labelling MRI and FDG-PET. *Neuroimage Clin.* 2017 Oct 31;17:405-414. doi: 10.1016/j.nicl.2017.10.033. PMID: 29159053; PMCID: PMC5683801.

[45] Fan AP, Khalighi MM, Guo J, Ishii Y, Rosenberg J, Wardak M, Park JH, Shen B, Holley D, Gandhi H, Haywood T, Singh P, Steinberg GK, Chin FT, Zaharchuk G. Identifying Hypoperfusion in Moyamoya Disease With Arterial Spin Labeling and an [15O]-Water Positron Emission Tomography/Magnetic Resonance Imaging Normative Database. *Stroke.* 2019 Feb;50(2):373-380. doi: 10.1161/STROKEAHA.118.023426. PMID: 30636572; PMCID: PMC7161423.

[46] Aizaz M, Moonen RPM, van der Pol JAJ, Prieto C, Botnar RM, Kooi ME. PET/MRI of atherosclerosis. *Cardiovasc Diagn Ther.* 2020 Aug;10(4):1120-1139. doi: 10.21037/cdt.2020.02.09. PMID: 32968664; PMCID: PMC7487378.

Chapter 5

MULTIPARAMETRIC MRI CHARACTERIZATION IN AUTISM SPECTRUM DISORDER

ABSTRACT

This study employed volumetry, cortical thickness and functional connectivity based on MRI data to improve characterization and prediction in autism spectrum disorders (ASD). Data from 127 children with ASD (13.5 ± 6.0 years) and 153 age- and gender-matched typically developing children (TD, 14.5 ± 5.7 years) were selected from the multi-center Functional Connectome Project. Regional gray matter volume and cortical thickness increased, whereas white matter volume decreased in ASD compared to TD children. Several disrupted functional connectivity of MRI (fcMRI) networks were also identified in ASD, including lower temporal, visual and superior frontal connectivity but higher inferior and dorsolateral prefrontal cortical fcMRI. Furthermore, volumetry and fcMRI were correlated with multiple clinical tests and phenotypic data, suggesting our imaging metrics could potentially serve as biomarkers in prognosis, diagnosis and disease progression monitoring.

Keywords: cortical thickness, volumetry, functional connectivity, phenotypic association, resting state fMRI, connectome, autism spectrum disorder

1. Introduction

Autism spectrum disorders (ASD) are a group of polygenetic developmental brain disorders with behavioral and cognitive impairment [1, 2]. Affected individuals exhibit stereotypical repetitive movements, restricted interests, lack of impulse control, speech deficits, impaired intelligence and social skills compared to typically developing (TD) children [3]. Several studies revealed both structural and functional connectivity deficits in ASD [4, 5]. Structural connectivity derived from diffusion tensor imaging in ASD children demonstrate increased diffusivity and/or reduced fractional anisotropy in the long occipitofrontal fasciculus and inter-hemispheric corpus callosal (e.g., minor and major forceps) commissure [6], asymmetric and under-connected arcuate fasciculus language pathways [7, 8], as well as reduced cerebellar-cortical interconnectivity [9]. Functional connectivity of MRI (fcMRI) shows abnormal disinhibition of some subcortical circuits [10], over- or under-connectivity in the superior temporal gyrus and amygdala [11].

A key clinical manifestation of ASD is impaired learning and social interactions [12]. Mirror mechanisms in frontoparietal and sensorimotor networks are involved in the imitation of others' actions in normal subjects [13], and have been suggested to be dysfunctional in children with ASD [14, 15]. In addition, neural networks underlying reflective mentalization [16] as well as emotional and interoceptive awareness [17] may be impaired in ASD. The inferior frontal gyrus (IFG), which is involved in high-level memory, language production and comprehension, and learning interactions [18-20], has been reported to be abnormal in ASD children. Within the IFG, the pars opercularis plays a role in social interactions including imitation control [21], while the pars triangularis is associated with language comprehension [22].

The goals of this study were: i) to evaluate multi-parametric functional and structural MRI of the brain changes in ASD versus TD children using small-worldness network analysis based on graph theory to derive local and global efficiency, and ii) using MRI/fMRI data to predict ASD clinical phenotypic outcomes, such as the revised autism diagnostic interview

(ADI-R), autism diagnostic observation schedule (ADOS), and intelligence quotient (IQ) scores reflecting different aspects of social and learning abilities of subjects [23].

2. METHODS

2.1. Participants and Phenotypic Information and MRI Imaging

Data was obtained from the multi-center Functional Connectome Project (FCP), which released MRI data of over 500 ASD patients (http://fcon_1000.projects.nitrc.org/indi/abide/). We downloaded the Autism Brain Imaging Data Exchange database from the COINS website (http://coins.mrn.org/) that hosted copies of data samples. In accordance with HIPAA guidelines and 1000 Functional Connectomes Project/INDI protocols, all datasets are anonymous, with no protected health information included. Consistent with the policies of the 1000 Functional Connectomes Project, data usage was approved for research purposes.

127 children with ASD (mean age: 13.5 ± 6.0 years, 24.1% of female), 153 age- and gender-matched control TD children (mean age: 14.5 ± 5.7 years, 24.8% of female) from the NYU/Yale/Stanford centers were selected for analyses based on age ranges. The full IQ scores were slightly lower in ASD group (104.3 ± 18.9) compared to TD group (111.7 ± 14.4), with P = 0.001. Imaging data consisted of high spatial resolution 3D T1-based MPRAGE sequence (image size = 160x256x256, resolution = 1x1x1mm^3) and resting-state (RS)-fMRI obtained using standard gradient echo EPI sequence (TR = 2000msec, resolution = 3x3x4mm^3, 180 volumes) with 33 slices covering the whole cerebrum [2].

The corresponding clinical data from five categories were also obtained, consisting of the ADOS scores, the ADI-R, and IQ tests (full scale and sub-functionality), social responsiveness scale (SRS) and Vinland adaptive behavior scale (VABS) with five domains. Detailed information regarding the phenotypic data was outlined in previously published articles [11, 12]. Briefly, the ADI-R is composed of 93 items focusing on the triadic functional domains, and administered via interview with categorical results provided. The full IQ tests consisted of verbal IQ (VIQ) and performance IQ (PIQ). The ADOS is a semi-structured assessment of social affection and communication behaviors, using four modules to account for individual expressive language level and chronological age. The SRS rating scale measures the social ability of ASD children (including total and subdomains of cognition, communication, awareness and motivation). The VABS instrument consists of social and personal skills for everyday living, including subdomains such as interpersonal empathy and socialization.

2.2. Image Processing and Data Analysis

2.2.1. Volumetry Analysis

Anatomical data were processed to derive the total supratentorial volume, regional subcortical volumes (45 regions), white matter (WM) volumes (70 regions), and cortical gray matter (GM) volumes (148 regions) using Freesurfer software (version 5.1.0) [24, 25]. Regional volume comparisons were implemented after supratentorial volume normalization. The cortical thickness of 148 cortical regions was measured automatically based on minimal communication distance between the gray and white matter ribbon of the projected cortical surface [26]. Cortical thickness measured with Freesurfer has been shown to be especially useful in characterizing the cortical folding and cytoarchitecture shaping in different age ranges [27].

2.2.2. fMRI Data Analysis

Quantitative fcMRI images and global quantitative values, as well as small-worldness analyses with volumetry, cortical thickness and fcMRI data, were derived based on the same processing methods described in previous chapters and in [2].

2.3. Correlational Analysis between Imaging and Phenotypic Data

Quantitative analysis of single imaging features of regional volume, N and Z from fcMRI, as well as the combined selected imaging features were correlated with the clinical data (i.e., ADOS, ADI-R, SRS, VABS, and IQ tests including both full and sub-domain scores). Bonferroni adjustment was implemented by multiplying the original p-values with both the number of category tests applied (x5 in this study) and the number of sub-domain tests (e.g., x10 for ADOS, x3 for IQ, x5 for ADI-R, x7 for SRS and x15 for VABS) of each category.

3. RESULTS

3.1. Volumetry Analysis

Volume and cortical thickness differences between the ASD and TD groups are shown in Figure 1. A particular finding is that the ASD group demonstrated significantly larger GM volume in the four brain lobes (with exception of the right medial orbital olfactory region) but less WM volume compared to the TD group, and the quantitative differences are listed in Table 1. Consistent with GM volumetric findings, the ASD group also showed significantly increased cortical thickness in all the four brain lobes, with a range of 2.8-5.2% increase at significance level of $P < 0.01$ [2].

3.2. fcMRI Analysis

With seeding in the caudate, the ASD children demonstrated reduced functional connectivity in the cingulum and middle temporal cortex compared to TD children, but increased connectivity in several regions including the inferior and dorsolateral frontal areas (Figure 2A). With seeding in the IFG pars triangularis, the ASD group showed reduced fcMRI of visual and temporal regions, but increased in the medial temporal areas (Figure 2B).

Table 1. Significant regional volume differences (P < 0.01) comparing children with autism spectrum disorder (ASD) to age-matched typically developing (TD) children after supratentorial volume normalization

Region and Location	V1- TD Children	V2- ASD Children	P value (**)	Percentage change % (Δ1)
Frontal GM				
Left inferior	0.852	0.938	0.0068	10.094%
Left superior	18.97	20.05	0.0010**	5.693%
Right superior	18.18	19.12	0.0034*	5.171%
Right medial orbital olfactory	1.204	1.104	0.0034*	-8.306%
Frontal WM–left lateral orbitofrontal	5.761	5.562	0.0090*	-3.454%
Occipital GM				
Left middle	4.941	5.292	0.0056*	7.104%
Left superior	2.623	2.902	0.0002**	10.637%
Right superior	3.279	3.582	0.0017*	9.241%
Parietal GM				
Left postcentral	3.961	4.230	0.0064	6.791%
Right superior	5.482	5.888	0.0054*	7.406%
Right postcentral	3.996	4.319	0.0020*	8.083%
Right precuneus	6.495	7.031	0.0006**	8.253%
Parietal WM				
Left postcentral	5.771	5.483	0.0074	-4.990%
Right supramarginal	7.791	7.410	0.0054*	-4.890%
Temporal WM				
Left fusiform	5.811	5.567	0.0085	-4.199%
Right inferior	5.157	4.890	0.0023*	-5.177%
Right superior	5.779	5.543	0.0058*	-4.084%

Note-Data (V1, V2) are mean brain volumes after normalization to the supratentorial volume with a scale factor of 1000, no unit.

** Calculated with two-sample t test to obtain original p-value (shown with P < 0.01 after Bonferroni adjustment) between two groups, and with Bonferroni multiple region correction (x8 factor given 4 brain lobes in two hemispheres).

* Indicates a significant difference with corrected P < 0.05 after Bonferroni adjustment.

Δ1 Indicates percentage change between volume of ASD children (V2) and volume of TD children (V1), calculated as Δ1 = (V2-V1)/V1*100%.

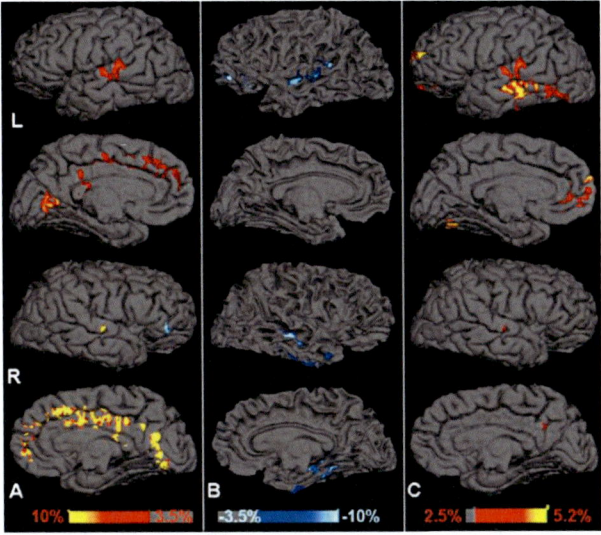

Figure 1. Regions with significant volume percentage increment (A, red color) in gray matter, and volume decrement in gray matter (only one small frontal cluster in blue) as well as white matter volume reduction (B, blue color) in autism compared to controls ($P < 0.01$). Significant cortical thickness increment in percentage change in autism compared to controls is shown in C with red color ($P < 0.01$). Both medial and lateral views on sagittal surface in the left and right hemispheres of an individual control subject are shown for gray matter volume (A), white matter volume (B) and cortical thickness (C) comparison between autistic children and controls. The percentage change of volume in autism was calculated as the mean difference between volumes of two groups normalized with individual supratentorial volume and scaled by the mean normalized volume of control group. Source Image: reference [2]; use with permission.

With seeding from IFG pars opercularis, the ASD group predominantly exhibited reduced functional connectivity with the superior frontal region (corrected $P < 0.05$; Figure 2C).

3.3. Correlation Analysis

The correlation analysis of the quantitative imaging features with phenotypic scores in ASD children, with both uncorrected and multiple-comparison corrected p-values was performed and results are listed in Table 2 [2].

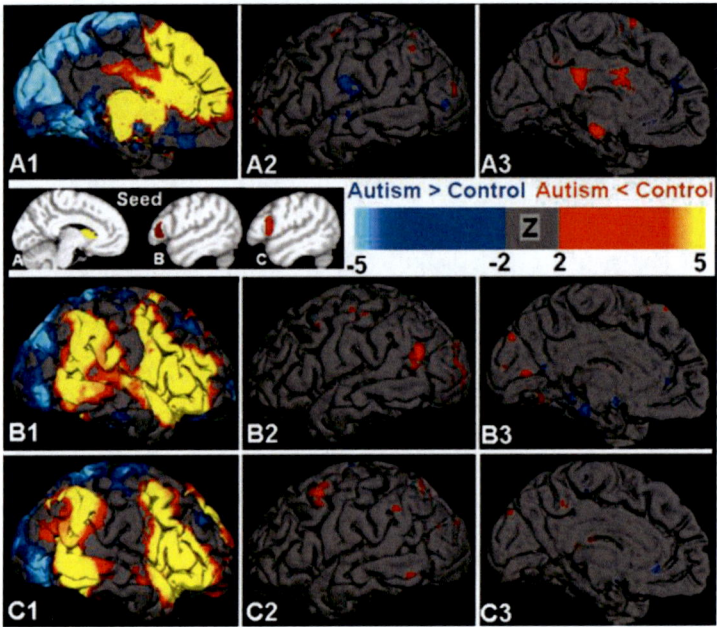

Figure 2. The functional connectivity network seeding from caudate and IFG region are demonstrated. In controls, the caudate-cortical network showed positive connections with the frontal and subcortical regions, and negative connections with the posterior visual and parietal areas (A1). The caudate-cortical network in children with ASD showed a primary reduction of cingulum and middle temporal connectivity (red color), but increased connectivity in several regions including the inferior and dorsolateral frontal areas (blue color, A2-A3). The functional connectivity network seeding from the IFG pars triangularis in controls (B1) showed positive connections with the frontal and temporal regions and negative connections with the posterior visual and superior parietal areas. Difference of connectivity pattern comparing autism to controls seeded from pars triangularis are shown in B2 and B3, with some reductions of visual and temporal connectivity in autism and increments in the regions including medial temporal areas (blue). Functional connectivity seeding from IFG pars opercularis is shown in C1-C3, with primarily decreased connectivity in autism in the superior frontal regions. Seed regions are shown in the upper left images, and all statistical results were obtained with the threshold of minimal $Z > 2.3$; cluster significance, $P < 0.05$, corrected. Source Image: reference [2]; use with permission.

Significant correlations were found: i) between the number of connections N based on fcMRI from the caudate and the full scale IQ in ASD children ($r = -0.47$, $P = 0.034$), ii) between caudate fcMRI N and ADOS scales ($r \leq -0.43$, $P < 0.005$), iii) between caudate fcMRI N and VABS social skill scores ($r = 0.35$, $P < 0.001$), iv) between caudate fcMRI

N and VABS interpersonal skills (r = -0.3, P < 0.001), v) between the caudate connectivity strength, Z score and the full scale IQ (r = -0.47, P = 0.034), vi) between caudate fcMRI Z and VABS scores (P < 0.001), vii) between the connections (both N and Z) from the two IFG seeds and ADOS tests (r ≤ -0.46, P ≤ 0.04), and viii) between the functional connections from the two IFG seeds and VABS scores (P < 0.001).

Table 2. Significant correlations between each single MRI quantitative metric and phenotypic tests in children with autism spectrum disorder (P < 0.05), adjusted with number of available patients for each test

MRI metric	Phenotypic Test	r	p
Caudate fcMRI (N)	ADOS social affection	-0.44	0.005
	ADOS research	-0.43	0.005
	VABS socialization	0.35	< 0.0001*
	VABS interpersonal skill	-0.30	< 0.0001*
	IQ (full)	-0.47	0.034
Caudate fcMRI (Z)	IQ (full)	-0.47	0.034
	VABS socialization	0.35	< 0.0001*
	VABS interpersonal skill	-0.44	< 0.0001*
	VABS daily living standard	0.26	0.0005*
IFG triangularis fcMRI (N)	ADOS module	-0.57	0.0016
	ADOS total	-0.46	0.014
	ADOS communication	-0.47	0.04
	ADOS research	-0.47	0.04
	VABS interpersonal skill	-0.43	< 0.0001*
IFG opercularis fcMRI (N)	ADOS module	-0.64	0.0002
IFG opercularis fcMRI (Z)	ADOS module	-0.50	0.007
	VABS socialization	0.34	0.0001*
	VABS interpersonal skill	-0.25	0.0006*

Note: N is the total number of voxels and Z is the average correlational z-value computed from the functional connectivity map (fcMRI) of each seed using a threshold of cluster corrected P < 0.05.

* Indicates a significant difference with corrected P < 0.05 after Bonferroni adjustment, with multiplication factors determined by both the number of category tests applied (x5 in this study) and the number of sub-domain tests (e.g., x10 for ADOS, x3 for IQ, x5 for ADI-R, x7 for SRS and x15 for VABS) of each category.

4. DISCUSSION

4.1. Brain Volume and Thickness Differences

Our findings of GM volume and cortical thickness increases but WM volume decreases in ASD compared to TD group were in general agreement with prior studies [28-30]. The increased cortical thickness in multiple regions throughout the cerebrum, together with decreased WM volumes in frontal and temporal regions, might represent a reduction in long-distance communication pathways with accompanying local GM volume increments. The small-worldness network analysis based on volumetry and fcMRI found no differences between ASD and TD children, while small-worldness analysis based on cortical thickness revealed reduced total and global efficiency in ASD [2]. As expected, both increased gray matter volume and cortical thickness in gray matter regions in ASD could lead to a reduction in global efficiency, consistent with EEG/MEG results [31, 32] that supported the hypothesis of unbalanced networks in autism [33].

4.2. Functional Connectivity Differences

Changes in caudate volume, caudate-cortical fcMRI, and IFG fcMRI were found to be highly predictive based on advanced machine learning algorithms. Most of the published literature on classification in autism was based on single imaging measures (such as volume, connectivity, or perfusion) [34-36]. The integrated multiparametric model demonstrates markedly improved accuracy (i.e., sensitivity and specificity) for classification (close to 100%) and prediction ($r > 0.94$) [2].

Consistent with task-based fMRI results [37, 38], we identified altered IFG functional connectivity, suggestive of deficit in the mirror mechanism in autistic children. DMN fcMRI disruption and altered interhemispheric functional connectivity were in agreement with previously reported studies in ASD [39, 40]. In addition, we found that caudate-cortical connectivity differed between ASD and TD children, and this metric correlated with full-scale IQ scores. A recent study reported aberrant functional connectivity from the caudate seed involving early developing brain areas, which implicated that developmental derangement of related functional brain circuits in ASD might begin at a young age (from 7-14 years old) [12]. Furthermore, small-worldness network analysis of fcMRI could not distinguish between ASD and TD groups, suggesting there was a functional compensatory mechanism in autism, including increased regional functional connectivity and reduced global, long-distance connectivity in ASD [2].

4.3. Other Considerations and Summary

The regional parcellation with Freesurfer used in our study had been shown to be a robust method. However, the results of direct volumetry and cortical thickness could be affected by the normalization errors of projecting individual brains to a template brain, given the younger age range of our subjects compared to the averaged template. Implementing spatial normalization with manual intervention and construction of age-specific templates in Freesurfer would be needed to help generalize the results to larger populations.

An additional limitation was that the clinical phenotypic scales were obtained in the first years of life of participants, and not necessarily the period during which they underwent MRI scanning. This might potentially increase the possibility of mismatch between symptoms and brain features.

In conclusion, largely increased GM volume and cortical thickness were found in ASD with decreased WM volume. Disrupted brain networks seeding from caudate and two orbitofrontal regions as well as DMN were identified in ASD as well. Moreover, the caudate volume, caudate-cortical fcMRI and IFG pars opercularis as well as triangularis fcMRI were highly predictive of phenotypic features in ASD. Our approach of analyzing the collective imaging features could potentially serve as imaging biomarkers in assessing disease prognosis and monitoring progression [2].

REFERENCES

[1] Rapin I, Tuchman RF. *Autism: definition, neurobiology, screening, diagnosis.* Pediatric clinics of North America. 2008;55(5):1129-46, viii.

[2] Zhou Y, Yu F, Duong T. Multiparametric MRI Characterization and Prediction in Autism Spectrum Disorder Using Graph Theory and Machine Learning. *PLoS ONE.* 2014;9(6):e90405.

[3] Kang S, O'Reilly M, Rojeski L, et al. Effects of tangible and social reinforcers on skill acquisition, stereotyped behavior, and task engagement in three children with autism spectrum disorders. *Res Dev Disabil.* 2013;34(2):739-44.

[4] Uddin LQ, Supekar K, Menon V. Reconceptualizing functional brain connectivity in autism from a developmental perspective. *Frontiers in Human Neuroscience.* 2013;7,458:1-11.

[5] Vissers ME, Cohen MX, Geurts HM. Brain connectivity and high functioning autism: A promising path of research that needs refined models, methodological convergence, and stronger behavioral link. *Neuroscience and Biobehavioral Reviews.* 2012;36:604-25.

[6] Travers BG, Adluru N, Ennis C, et al. Diffusion tensor imaging in autism spectrum disorder: a review. Autism Res. 2012;5(5):289-313.

[7] Lange N, Dubray MB, Lee JE, et al. Atypical diffusion tensor hemispheric asymmetry in autism. *Autism Res.* 2010;3(6):350-8.

[8] Fletcher PT, Whitaker RT, Tao R, et al. Microstructural connectivity of the arcuate fasciculus in adolescents with high-functioning autism. *NeuroImage.* 2010;51(3):1117-25.

[9] Sivaswamy L, Kumar A, Rajan D, et al. A diffusion tensor imaging study of the cerebellar pathways in children with autism spectrum disorder. *J Child Neurol.* 2010;25(10):1223-31.

[10] Langen M, Schnack HG, Nederveen H, et al. Changes in the developmental trajectories of striatum in autism. *Biological psychiatry.* 2009;66(4):327-33.

[11] Di Martino A, Kelly C, Grzadzinski R, et al. Aberrant striatal functional connectivity in children with autism. *Biol Psychiatry.* 2011;69(9):847-56.

[12] Di Martino A, Ross K, Uddin LQ, Sklar AB, Castellanos FX, Milham MP. Functional brain correlates of social and nonsocial processes in autism spectrum disorders: an activation likelihood estimation meta-analysis. *Biol Psychiatry.* 2009;65(1):63-74.

[13] Hamilton AF. Reflecting on the mirror neuron system in autism: a systematic review of current theories. *Dev Cogn Neurosci.* 2013;3:91-105.

[14] Gallese V, Rochat MJ, Berchio C. The mirror mechanism and its potential role in autism spectrum disorder. *Developmental Medicine & Child Neurology* 2012;55:15-22.

[15] Rizzolatti G, Febbri-Destro M. Mirror neurons: from discovery to autism. *Exp Brain Res.* 2003;2010(200):223-37.

[16] Frith U. Mind blindness and the brain in autism. *Neuron.* 2001;32:969-79.

[17] Ebisch SJ, Gallese V, Willems RM, et al. Altered intrinsic functional connectivity of anterior and posterior insula regions in high-functioning participants with autism spectrum disorder. *Human Brain Mapping.* 2011;32(7):1013-28.

[18] Greenlee JD, Oya H, Kawasaki H, et al. Functional connections within the human inferior frontal gyrus. *J Comp Neurol.* 2007;503(4):550-9.

[19] Nixon P, Lazarova J, Hodinott-Hill I, Gough P, Passingham R. The inferior frontal gyrus and phonological processing: an investigation using rTMS. *J Cogn Neurosci.* 2004;16(2):289-300.

[20] Hsieh L, Gandour J, Wong D, Hutchins GD. Functional heterogeneity of inferior frontal gyrus is shaped by linguistic experience. *Brain Lang.* 2001;76(3):227-52.

[21] Rudie JD, Shehzad Z, Hernandez LM, et al. Reduced functional integration and segregation of distributed neural systems underlying social and emotional information processing in autism spectrum disorders. *Cereb Cortex*; 22(5):1025-37.

[22] Geva S, Jones PS, Crinion JT, Price CJ, Baron JC, Warburton EA. The neural correlates of inner speech defined by voxel-based lesion-symptom mapping. *Brain*;134(Pt 10):3071-82.

[23] Buitelaar JK, van der Wees M, Swaab-Barneveld H, van der Gagg RJ. Verbal memory and performance IQ predict theory of mind and emotion recognition ability in children with autistic spectrum disorders and in psychiatric control children. *J Child Psychol Psychiatry*. 1999;40(6):869-81.

[24] Zhou Y. *Functional and Neuroimaging Methods and Frontiers*. Nova Science Publishers. 2018.

[25] Fischl B. FreeSurfer. *Neuroimage*. 2012;62(2):774-81.

[26] Fischl B, Dale AM. Measuring the thickness of the human cerebral cortex from magnetic resonance images. *Proc Natl Acad Sci U S A*. 2000;97(20):11050-5.

[27] Sowell ER, Peterson BS, Kan E, et al. Sex differences in cortical thickness mapped in 176 healthy individuals between 7 and 87 years of age. *Cereb Cortex*. 2007;17(7):1550-60.

[28] Ecker C, Ginestet C, Feng Y, et al. Brain surface anatomy in adults with autism: the relationship between surface area, cortical thickness, and autistic symptoms. *JAMA Psychiatry*. 2013;70(1):59-70.

[29] Ecker C, Stahl D, Daly E, Johnston P, Thomson A, Murphy DG. Is there a common underlying mechanism for age-related decline in cortical thickness? *Neuroreport*. 2009;20(13):1155-60.

[30] Hardan AY, Muddasani S, Vemulapalli M, Keshavan MS, Minshew NJ. An MRI study of increased cortical thickness in autism. *Am J Psychiatry*. 2006;163(7):1290-2.

[31] Khan S, Gramfort A, Shetty NR, et al. Local and long-range functional connectivity is reduced in concert in autism spectrum disorders. *Proc Natl Acad Sci U S A*. 2013;110(8):3107-12.

[32] Peters JM, Taquet M, Vega C, et al. Brain functional networks in syndromic and non-syndromic autism: a graph theoretical study of EEG connectivity. *BMC Med*. 2013;11(1):54.

[33] Walsh CA, Morrow EM, Rubenstein JL. Autism and brain development. *Cell*. 2008;135(3):396-400.

[34] van der Zande FH, Hofman PA, Backes WH. Mapping hypercapnia-induced cerebrovascular reactivity using BOLD MRI. *Neuroradiology.* 2005;47(2):114-20.

[35] Wang H, Chen C, Fushing H. Extracting multiscale pattern information of fMRI based functional brain connectivity with application on classification of autism spectrum disorders. *PLoS One.* 2012;7(10):e45502.

[36] Duchesnay E, Cachia A, Boddaert N, et al. Feature selection and classification of imbalanced datasets Application to PET images of children with autistic spectrum disorders. *NeuroImage.* 2011;57:1003-14.

[37] Villalobos ME, Mizuno A, Dahl BC, Kemmotsu N, Muller RA. Reduced functional connectivity between V1 and inferior frontal cortex associated with visuomotor performance in autism. *Neuroimage.* 2005;25(3):916-25.

[38] Lee PS, Yerys BE, Della Rosa A, et al. Functional connectivity of the inferior frontal cortex changes with age in children with autism spectrum disorders: a fcMRI study of response inhibition. *Cereb Cortex.* 2009;19(8):1787-94.

[39] Anderson JS, Druzgal TJ, Froehlich A, et al. Decreased interhemispheric functional connectivity in autism. *Cereb Cortex.* 2011;21(5):1134-46.

[40] Assaf M, Jagannathan K, Calhoun VD, et al. Abnormal functional connectivity of default mode sub-networks in autism spectrum disorder patients. *Neuroimage.* 2010;53(1):247-56.

ABOUT THE AUTHOR

Yongxia Zhou is a medical imaging scientist, specialized in neuroimaging and neurosciences applications. She had completed her PhD degree from University of Southern California in Biomedical imaging in 2004 and had been trained and worked as neuroimaging scientists in several prestigious institutes including Columbia University, New York University and University of Pennsylvania and NIH. Her research focuses on multi modal neuroimaging including MRI/PET and EEG/MEG instrumentation as well as the integration of these multi-modal to make the best usage of each modality and to help interpreting underlying co-existing pathophysiological for better disease diagnosis and treatment. Her specific interests in MRI technology include brain mapping of blood flow, oxygen saturation and extraction fraction and metabolism as well as brain network assessment with advanced fMRI activity/connectivity methods and PET/MRI confirmation. Applications of these comprehensive techniques in multiple domains including memory and cognition, neurodegenerative diseases such as dementia and brain injury are the main focus. She has published more than 10 books and 5 book chapters, 100 papers and abstracts in well-known international journals and conferences. She has also served as several journals, books and international conference editor and reviewer including *JMRI*, *RSNA*, *HBM*, *AJNR*, *PlosOne*, *ISMRM* and *ICAD*.

INDEX

#

9-[18F]fluoropropyl-(+)-dihydrotetrabenazine, 48

A

abrupt motion artifact, 32
absolute clustering coefficient, 12
absolute local efficiency, 27, 87, 88, 123
accuracy (ACC), xi, xiii, 2, 4, 12, 29, 30, 32, 33, 34, 63, 70, 93, 127, 135, 146
ADNI database, 5, 48, 71, 108
advanced imaging technique, xi, xv, 33, 105, 107, 108
affective disorders, 53, 61
affective mentalizing, 70, 97
age, xvi, 5, 6, 72, 109, 125, 137, 139, 140, 142, 147, 150, 151
age-matched, 5, 142
aging brain, 54, 109
Aging Brain with Vasculature, Ischemia and Behavior (ABVIB), xi, 109
aging effect, 116, 120, 125
Alzheimer's disease neuroimaging initiative (ADNI), x, 5, 6, 34, 35, 48, 71, 72, 108, 109
amygdala, viii, 16, 47, 76, 90, 91, 114, 122, 124, 138
amyloid, ix, xiv, 55, 56, 67, 68, 69, 71, 72, 73, 74, 75, 89, 94, 107, 121, 122, 128, 130
amyloid accumulation, ix, 56, 68, 72, 73, 74, 89
amyloid burden, 55, 74, 75, 122
amyloid deposition, 55, 56
Analysis of Functional NeuroImages (AFNI), 73
angular, 70, 92
angular gyrus, 70
anterior cingulate, 10, 17, 18, 47, 70, 92, 93, 107
anterior putamen, 47, 49, 50
anterior temporal cortex, 114, 122, 124
anterior thalamic radiation, 110, 116, 118, 119, 125
anterior thalamic radiation tract, 125
anxiety, vii, 46, 47, 58, 59
apathy, vii, 46, 47, 58, 68, 69, 92, 94, 107
arcuate fasciculus, viii, 138, 148

area under curve (AUC), 93
arterial spin labeling (ASL), 57, 58, 93, 99, 101, 127, 136
atrophy, vii, viii, xiii, xiv, 1, 2, 4, 6, 13, 15, 30, 33, 45, 53, 57, 68, 70, 73, 74, 89, 90, 91, 92, 93, 100, 106, 107, 109, 111, 112, 113, 121, 122, 124, 125, 126, 128, 133, 134
attention, viii, 4, 7, 68, 69, 76, 78, 122, 125
attention deficits, 125
attentional deficit, 31
attentional network, xii, 1, 2, 4, 69, 70, 80, 90
attentional network deficits, xii, 4
auditory, xi, xiii, 2, 9, 10, 17, 18, 31, 32, 34
auditory cortex, 10, 17
auditory network, xi, xiii, 2, 17, 18, 31, 34
autism diagnostic observation schedule (ADOS), 139, 141, 144, 145
autism spectrum disorders (ASD), viii, x, xii, xvi, 137, 138, 139, 140, 141, 142, 143, 144, 146, 147, 148, 149, 150, 151
autistic children, ix, 143, 146
AV-133, 47, 48, 50
axial diffusivity (AD), 5, 47, 48, 56, 59, 69, 70, 71, 92, 102, 108, 110, 111, 116, 117, 118, 119, 120, 122, 125, 127, 130, 133
axonal degeneration, viii, ix, xii, 106, 107, 116, 118, 119, 125

B

basal forebrain, 2
basal ganglia, vii, xi, xiii, 2, 10, 13, 14, 15, 16, 17, 18, 19, 20, 22, 30, 31, 32, 33, 36, 41, 46, 47, 53, 54, 75, 76, 80, 81, 90, 113, 114, 121, 122, 124, 127, 128
basal ganglia network, 3, 10, 32, 41
baseline, xii, xv, 67, 71, 72, 73, 76, 77, 78, 79, 80, 81, 82, 83, 87, 90, 91, 92, 109, 120

baseline-longitudinal comparison, xii, 71
behavior variant (bv), vii, xiv, 67, 68, 72
behavioral deficits, xiv, 67, 71
behavioral symptoms, 68
behavioral variant frontotemporal dementia (bvFTD), vii, xii, xiv, 67, 68, 69, 70, 71, 72, 75, 76, 77, 79, 82, 84, 86, 92, 93, 94, 95, 96, 97, 99, 100, 101, 106, 122
better diagnosis, 56
betweenness centrality (BC), 11, 94, 95, 151
biological factor, xi, xiv, 46, 56
biological factor characterization, xiv, 46
biological factor investigation, xi, 56
biomarkers, xii, xvi, 33, 43, 57, 60, 101, 137
blind source separation, 9
blood flow, 36, 47, 58, 108, 127, 130, 133, 153
Bonferroni adjustment, 141, 142, 145
bradykinesia, 46
brain abnormalities, xii, xiii, 1, 69
brain architecture, 92
brain atrophy, ix, xi, xiv, xv, 2, 7, 35, 57, 67, 71, 89, 93, 94, 105, 127
brain circuit, ix, x, xi, xiii, xv, 2, 32, 33, 47, 68, 90, 94, 128, 147
brain clusters, 14, 113
brain function, 4, 11, 31, 53, 56, 110, 125, 150
brain hubs, 10
brain morphology, xv, 105, 108
brain networks, vii, xiv, 3, 32, 33, 42, 67, 69, 71, 100
brain reserve, 54, 90
brain science, x, xi, xiv, 45, 54, 56
brain status switching, 32
brain stem, xv, 67, 72, 73, 77, 81, 83, 84, 85, 113, 114
brain structure, v, 40, 43, 105, 109
bvFTD, vii, xii, xiv, 67, 68, 69, 70, 71, 72, 75, 76, 77, 79, 82, 84, 86, 92, 93, 94, 106, 122

bvFTD patients, xiv, 67, 69, 70, 71, 75, 76, 77, 86, 92, 93, 94

C

calcarine, 10, 15, 17, 56, 76, 78, 90, 116, 122
caregiver burden, 106, 128
caudate, ix, xi, xiv, 8, 10, 14, 15, 17, 18, 19, 24, 25, 32, 45, 46, 47, 48, 49, 50, 51, 52, 74, 75, 76, 78, 90, 115, 121, 122, 124, 126, 141, 144, 145, 146, 147
causal factor, 108
central executive-function network (CEN), 126
central nervous system, 48
central opercular cortex, 92
centrum semiovale, 126
cerebellar-cortical interconnectivity, viii, 138
cerebellum, ix, xiii, xv, 2, 3, 10, 13, 15, 17, 18, 20, 30, 33, 48, 51, 56, 61, 67, 74, 75, 76, 78, 79, 80, 81, 83, 90, 94, 114, 116, 121, 122, 124, 127
cerebral blood flow, 56, 63
cerebral peduncle, 7, 13, 76, 77, 122
cerebrospinal fluid (CSF), 7, 48, 60
cerebrovascular disease, 109, 132, 134
cingulum, vii, xvi, 69, 105, 106, 110, 112, 113, 116, 118, 119, 120, 122, 124, 127, 141, 144
cingulum bundle, 112
classification, xiii, 1, 5, 12, 29, 33, 93, 101, 126, 146, 151
classification accuracy, 126
classification evaluation, xiii, 1, 5
classifier performance, 12
clinical data, ix, 5, 127, 139, 141
clinical diagnosis, 93
clinical disease severity, 69
clinical impairments, vii, 68

clinical manifestation, 138
clinical outcome, 54, 61
clinical phenotypic outcomes, 138
clinical symptom, 2, 7, 53
clinical tests, xii, xvi, 137
closing eyes, x, xii, xv, 67, 71, 76, 78, 84, 85, 86, 87, 88, 90, 91, 94, 122
cluster level, 8, 11
cluster size, 14, 113, 114
cluster-corrected, 9, 76, 77
clustering coefficient (CC), 11, 47, 63, 98, 127
cognitive dysfunction, 4
cognitive function, 60, 116, 119
cognitive impairment, viii, 5, 36, 39, 40, 42, 48, 71, 106, 108, 125, 129, 130, 131, 132, 133, 134, 135, 138
combined MRI/PET, 128
communicating, 7
communication, 31, 32, 115, 140, 145, 146
compensation, ix, x, xv, 29, 31, 32, 54, 67, 90, 91, 94, 124
compensation roles, 90
compensation strategy, x
compensatory mechanism, 3, 70, 147
compensatory role, 3
comprehensive analysis, xiii, 1
conductivity, ix, x, xiv, 34, 45, 53, 73, 76, 78, 89, 94, 121, 122, 128
connectivity deficits, viii, ix, xv, 105, 115, 124, 127, 138
connectome, xvi, 137, 139
conventional low frequency band, x, xv, 105, 124
conventional RSFC, 10, 88
coordination dysfunction, 54
corpus callosum, 76, 77, 89, 93, 106, 112, 122, 124, 125
correlation analysis, 42, 143
correlation matrix, 11
correlational quantification, xiii, 1, 5, 8
cortical folding, 140

cortical thickness, x, xii, xvi, 92, 93, 137, 140, 141, 143, 146, 147, 150
corticospinal tract, xii, xvi, 105, 106, 110, 112, 116, 118, 119, 120, 122, 124, 127
corticostriatal, vii, 3, 9, 10, 17, 31, 32
corticostriatal and prefrontal connectivity, 32
corticostriatal loop, vii, 3
corticostriatal network, 10, 17, 31
cross-sectional comparison, 76, 90
cross-validation (CV), xi, 12, 33, 57, 102
cuneal, 69
cuneus, 10, 17, 76, 78, 122
cytoarchitecture shaping, 140

D

data cohort, ix, xv, 6, 17, 35, 68, 72, 105, 109, 127
deep brain stimulation (DBS), 53, 54, 61, 62
default mode network, vii, xiii, 2, 3, 8, 19, 69, 126
default mode network (DMN), vii, xi, xiii, 2, 3, 4, 8, 10, 17, 18, 19, 24, 26, 27, 31, 32, 34, 69, 70, 81, 83, 85, 86, 91, 121, 122, 126, 146, 147
deformation based morphometry, 92, 100
demographic information, 6, 72, 109
demyelination, ix, xii, xvi, 106, 107, 116, 118, 119, 124, 125, 127
dependency, viii, 106
dependent group, x, xii, xv, 105, 109, 111, 112, 113, 114, 115, 116, 118, 120, 123, 124, 125, 127, 128
dependent living, xii, xv, 105, 106, 108, 116, 119
dependent participants, ix, 112, 113, 116, 119
depression, vii, 43, 46, 47, 53, 54, 58, 59, 62, 108, 132
depression symptom, 47, 54, 59

depressive symptoms, 107
detection sensitivity, 10
diagnosis, x, xii, xvi, 36, 39, 58, 59, 68, 93, 94, 95, 128, 129, 137, 148
diagnostic criteria, 95, 106, 129
diffuse WM abnormalities, 107
diffusion directions, 73, 110
diffusion tensor imaging (DTI), ix, x, xi, xii, xiii, xiv, 1, 2, 6, 13, 30, 33, 40, 52, 67, 71, 72, 73, 89, 91, 102, 106, 107, 109, 110, 111, 112, 116, 118, 120, 121, 122, 125, 133, 138, 148
diffusivity metrics, xii, xv, 105, 108, 110
direct MRI-based targeting (dTM), 54
disability, viii, 53, 106, 107, 108, 127, 132
discoordination, ix, 67, 124
disease abnormalities, xi, xiii, 2, 34
disease classification, 30, 70
disease diagnosis, x, 127, 153
disease heterogeneity, 3
disease mechanism, x, xii, 46, 93, 127
disease progression, xii, xvi, 53, 69, 90, 116, 120, 125, 137
disease severity, xii, xvi, 31, 106, 108, 128
disease-specific, x
disinhibition, viii, 68, 69, 90, 92, 107, 116, 119, 124, 125, 131, 138
disinhibition behavior, 116, 119, 125
disinhibition function, 90
disrupted brain networks, 31, 147
DLPFC, 3, 4, 10, 17, 18
dominant hemisphere, 92, 99
dopamine, vii, ix, xi, xiv, 3, 45, 46, 47, 49, 50, 52, 53, 54, 57, 59, 60, 61, 121, 128
dopamine deficiency, 53
dopamine denervation, 48
dopamine depletion, 54, 61
dopamine neurons, 53
dopamine release, 46
dopamine storage, ix, xiv, 45, 52
dopamine transmitter, vii, 46

dopamine transporter (DAT), ix, xi, xiv, 45, 46, 47, 48, 49, 50, 52, 53, 57, 59, 121
dopaminergic neuron, xiv, 3, 45, 47, 52
dopaminergic treatment, 53
dorsal attentional network (DAN), 4, 10, 17, 18, 19, 22, 32, 69, 74, 75, 76, 85, 86, 122, 124
dorsal putamen (DPU), 47
dorsolateral attentional network, 2, 69, 80, 90
dorsolateral prefrontal cortex (DLPFC), viii, xiii, 2, 3, 4, 10, 13, 15, 17, 18, 22, 30, 33, 54, 69, 74, 75, 80, 82, 83, 85, 91, 116, 121, 122
DR components, 10, 19, 20, 21, 22, 83, 84, 86, 87, 115, 117
dual regression (DR), viii, xi, xiii, 1, 2, 4, 9, 10, 17, 18, 19, 20, 21, 22, 23, 24, 31, 33, 39, 52, 60, 68, 79, 80, 81, 83, 84, 86, 87, 90, 96, 110, 115, 117, 121
dual regression (ICA-DR), viii, x, xi, xiii, xiv, xv, 1, 2, 4, 9, 10, 17, 18, 19, 20, 21, 22, 23, 24, 32, 33, 39, 52, 67, 68, 71, 74, 77, 79, 80, 81, 82, 84, 85, 86, 87, 90, 96, 110, 121, 122, 124, 128
dynamic correlation, 70

E

early onset of AD (EOAD), 93
early prevention, 3, 33
EEG, 70, 98, 146, 150, 153
EEG/MEG, 146, 153
effective treatment, x
efficiency, x, xiii, xv, 2, 4, 11, 12, 27, 29, 33, 34, 54, 68, 86, 87, 88, 91, 92, 105, 106, 118, 121, 122, 123, 124, 127, 128, 138, 146
efficiency analysis, x
emotion, vii, 32, 68, 116, 119, 125, 150
emotional and interoceptive awareness, 138

episodic memory, 126
excessive motion, 7, 74
executive dysfunction, vii, 4
executive function, vii, 4, 32, 37, 68, 69, 114, 116, 119, 125, 133
eyes closing, 68, 73, 82, 88, 89, 91
eyes opening, 68, 73, 77, 85, 86, 88, 89

F

factional amplitude of low frequency fluctuation (fALFF), ix, xiii, xv, 2, 8, 9, 12, 23, 25, 26, 27, 28, 30, 32, 34, 69, 74, 88, 105, 110, 118, 121, 122, 123, 124, 126
fast reconstruction, 57
FDG glucose, ix, 67, 72, 75, 76
flip angle, 6, 73, 109
fluoxetine, 54
fMRI activation, 126
FMRIB Software Library (FSL), 7, 8, 73, 110
forceps major, 110
forceps minor, 110
four brain lobes, x, 9, 141
fractional amplitude of low frequency fluctuation, ix, xiii, 2, 106
fractional amplitude of low frequency fluctuation (fALFF), ix, xiii, xv, 2, 8, 9, 12, 23, 25, 26, 27, 28, 30, 32, 34, 69, 74, 88, 105, 106, 110, 118, 121, 122, 123, 124, 126
fractional anisotropy (FA), viii, ix, xii, xv, 7, 13, 30, 61, 73, 76, 77, 89, 92, 93, 105, 106, 107, 110, 111, 112, 117, 120, 121, 122, 124, 125, 127, 138
frame displacement (FD), 7, 12, 13, 32, 74
free water, 107, 131
Freesurfer software, 140
frontal, vii, ix, xi, xii, xiii, xiv, 2, 3, 4, 8, 9, 10, 14, 16, 17, 18, 20, 21, 24, 25, 30, 31,

32, 34, 45, 49, 51, 52, 53, 54, 55, 68, 70, 74, 75, 76, 78, 80, 90, 92, 93, 106, 107, 112, 113, 114, 115, 121, 122, 124, 125, 126, 128, 141, 142, 143, 144, 146, 151
frontal eye field (FEF), 8, 24, 25
frontal lobe, 92, 93, 107
frontal network, 9, 10, 17, 20, 21
frontal pole, 14, 114, 122, 126
frontal WM lesion, 107
fronto-insular, 69, 70, 92
frontoinsular connectivity, 70
frontoparietal and sensorimotor networks, 138
frontoparietal network (FPN), vii, xi, xii, xiii, 2, 4, 10, 17, 18, 19, 31, 32, 33, 34, 69, 70, 81, 115, 122
fronto-temporal circuit, 92
frontotemporal dementia (FTD), vii, viii, x, xi, xiv, 57, 63, 67, 68, 69, 70, 72, 73, 74, 75, 76, 77, 78, 79, 81, 82, 83, 84, 85, 86, 87, 88, 89, 91, 92, 93, 94, 95, 96, 97, 98, 99, 100, 101, 102, 103, 121, 122, 128, 131, 135
frontotemporal hypometabolism, 93
frontotemporal lobar degeneration neuroimaging initiative (NIFD), xi, 72, 100
frontotemporal regions, 89
FTD patients, ix, x, xi, xv, 67, 68, 69, 71, 72, 73, 74, 75, 76, 77, 78, 79, 81, 82, 83, 84, 85, 86, 87, 88, 89, 91, 94
full IQ scores, 139
functional brain networks, 41, 42, 126
functional compensation, xi, xiii, 2, 18, 27, 31, 34, 86
functional connectivity, viii, ix, xi, xii, xiii, xiv, xv, xvi, 2, 3, 4, 6, 7, 8, 12, 18, 19, 23, 24, 27, 31, 33, 36, 37, 38, 41, 42, 45, 52, 53, 54, 67, 70, 71, 77, 79, 80, 81, 83, 84, 85, 86, 90, 92, 96, 97, 100, 103, 105, 110, 115, 116, 121, 122, 124, 126, 127, 134, 137, 138, 141, 143, 144, 145, 146, 149, 150, 151
functional connectivity of MRI (fcMRI), viii, x, xvi, 7, 8, 9, 11, 53, 54, 90, 137, 138, 140, 141, 142, 144, 145, 146, 147, 151
Functional Connectome Project (FCP), xi, xvi, 137, 139
functional coordination, xiii, 1, 14, 15, 31, 114
functional dysconnectivity, ix, xv, 67
functional MRI (fMRI), vii, ix, xii, xv, 1, 3, 4, 5, 6, 11, 27, 29, 33, 36, 37, 39, 42, 46, 52, 67, 68, 69, 71, 72, 73, 85, 91, 95, 97, 98, 102, 107, 109, 110, 115, 117, 125, 126, 130, 134, 137, 138, 139, 140, 151, 153
fusiform, 14, 15, 55, 79, 80, 90, 121, 126, 142

G

gender, xvi, 46, 55, 63, 72, 109, 137, 139
gender differences, 46, 55
genetics, 93
genu of corpus callosum, 76, 77, 89, 122
global, ix, xiii, xv, 2, 4, 8, 11, 12, 23, 24, 25, 26, 27, 28, 29, 33, 34, 54, 70, 86, 87, 88, 89, 91, 92, 105, 118, 122, 123, 124, 126, 138, 140, 146, 147
global efficiency, x, xiii, 2, 4, 11, 12, 29, 33, 34, 54, 86, 87, 92, 118, 122, 138, 146
global RSFC, 12
global VMHC, xiii, 2, 8, 12, 23, 24, 26, 33, 34
globus pallidus, 3
glucose hypometabolism, ix, 94
glucose metabolism, 63, 68, 72, 75, 100
GPD patients, xiii, 1, 6, 13, 15, 30, 33, 49, 50
gradient-echo EPI, 6, 73, 109

gradual progression, 68
graph theory, x, xiii, 1, 4, 9, 11, 69, 70, 86, 98, 110, 138, 148
gray matter (GM), x, xii, xiii, xiv, xvi, 1, 2, 6, 7, 8, 13, 15, 30, 33, 37, 45, 53, 54, 55, 56, 57, 61, 63, 68, 70, 73, 74, 92, 93, 106, 107, 109, 112, 113, 121, 122, 124, 125, 126, 137, 140, 141, 142, 143, 146, 147
gray matter atrophy, xiii, xiv, 1, 2, 6, 13, 15, 30, 33, 45, 53, 57, 68, 70, 73, 74, 93, 106, 109, 112, 113, 125
gray matter density, 7, 14, 15, 55, 56, 92, 93, 107, 112, 113, 124, 126
gray matter volume, x, xii, xvi, 137, 143, 146
group ICA, 9

H

hallucinations, 4, 40
Hayling test scores, 107
healthy controls (HC), 41, 42, 47, 49, 51, 52, 100
high correlations, xi, xiii, 2, 34
high spatiotemporal resolution, 56
hippocampal formation, 8
hippocampus, viii, 14, 16, 18, 55, 75, 76, 78, 79, 81, 89, 90, 107, 110, 122
hippocampus connection, 110
hybrid ICA, 9, 10
hybrid PET/MRI, 46
hyper-connectivity, xi, xiii, 2, 3, 20, 22, 31, 32, 33, 34
hyper-connectivity pattern, 31, 32
hyperorality, 68
hyper-synchronization, 3
hyper-synchrony, 107
hypo-connectivity, 22
hypometabolism, vii, xv, 57, 67, 68, 75, 76, 89, 90, 92, 93, 122, 128

hypoperfusion, 47, 57, 69, 92, 93, 136
hypothalamus, 8, 14, 15, 16, 18, 30, 76, 78, 80, 81, 90, 91, 114, 115, 121, 122, 124

I

ICA decomposition, 10, 17
ICA-DR, viii, x, xi, xiii, xiv, xv, 2, 9, 10, 17, 18, 21, 22, 32, 33, 67, 71, 74, 77, 79, 80, 81, 82, 84, 85, 86, 87, 90, 121, 122, 124, 128
ICA-DR model, 10
ICA-DR network connectivity, 32
imaging abnormalities, xi, xii, xiv, 94
imaging biomarkers, v, xi, xiii, 2, 34, 46, 58, 64, 67, 147
imaging evidence, ix, 69, 94
imaging hallmarks, viii, 3, 107
imitation control, 138
impaired intelligence, viii, 138
impaired performance, 30
impulse control, 41, 47, 59, 60
impulse control disorder (ICD), 41, 47, 53, 59, 60
impulsivity control, 32
increased diffusivity, viii, 116, 119, 138
independent component analysis (ICA), viii, x, xi, xiii, xiv, xv, 1, 2, 3, 4, 9, 10, 17, 18, 21, 22, 31, 32, 33, 39, 67, 68, 69, 70, 71, 74, 77, 79, 80, 81, 82, 84, 85, 86, 87, 90, 92, 97, 110, 115, 117, 121, 122, 124, 128
independent component analysis with dual regression (ICA-DR), viii, x, xi, xiii, xiv, xv, 2, 9, 10, 17, 18, 21, 22, 32, 33, 67, 71, 74, 77, 79, 80, 81, 82, 84, 85, 86, 87, 90, 121, 122, 124, 128
independent group, xv, 105, 113, 114, 115, 116, 117, 118, 119, 120, 122, 123, 124, 125, 127
independent living, xii, xv, 105, 108, 112, 114, 115

independent participants, ix, xv, 105, 112, 113, 114, 116, 118, 123, 127
individual variability, 3, 38
inertia, 68
inferior frontal gyrus (IFG), 70, 138, 142, 143, 144, 145, 146, 147, 149
inferior fronto-occipital fasciculus, 106, 110, 116, 118, 119, 124
inferior longitudinal fasciculus, 110
inferior parietal cortex, 81, 83, 91
inferior parietal lobe, 10, 17
inferior temporal cortex, 15, 126
inferior temporal gyrus, 14, 91, 92
information processing, 7, 124, 149
information processing speed, 124
inhibition, xii, xvi, 69, 105, 125, 127, 131, 151
inhibitory functioning, 107
initial visit, 116, 117, 120, 125
insula, 2, 3, 10, 13, 15, 17, 30, 69, 91, 92, 99, 149
insular, xii, 2, 4, 18, 22, 31, 32, 33, 56, 74, 75, 76, 78, 81, 83, 84, 85, 86, 89, 90, 91, 92, 94, 121, 122, 126
insular network, 4
insular-DAN, 22, 31
insular-DMN, 23, 31
integrated multiparametric model, 146
integrated PET/MRI, viii, xi, xiv, 46, 56
integrated PET/MRI modalities, 56
intelligence quotient (IQ), 139, 141, 144, 145, 147, 150
inter- DMN and DAN, 84, 91, 94
interhemispheric coordination, xi, xiii, xiv, 1, 4, 14, 15, 33, 45, 52, 114
interhemispheric correlation, ix, 15, 76, 94
interhemispheric functional coordination, 7
internal capsule, 76, 77, 89, 122
inter-network, ix, x, xi, xiii, 4, 10, 17, 18, 23, 31, 32, 77
inter-network connectivity patterns, 31
inter-network coordination, 11
inter-network correlation, x, 17
inter-network modulation, ix
inter-network remapping, 18, 77
interval, 73, 82, 83, 87, 91
intra- and inter- network connectivity, 10, 79, 115
intra- and inter- network dysconnectivity, 94
intra- and inter-network, viii, 1, 4, 10, 17, 34, 36, 82
intracalcarine cortex, 69
intrahemispheric connectivity, 92
intra-network, 4, 8, 10, 33
intra-network connectivity, 10
intra-parietal sulcus, 8
intrinsic network remapping, xiii, 1, 4
Ioflupane, 47
ischemic pathology, 126

K

k-means nearest-neighbor (KNN), 12, 29

L

lack of impulse control, viii, 138
language, viii, 114, 115, 116, 119, 124, 138, 140
language comprehension, 138
language production and comprehension, 138
L-DOPA treatment, 53
learning and memory, 53, 116, 119, 125
learning interactions, 138
left frontoparietal network, 70
leukoaraiosis, 126, 133
levodopa (L-DOPA), 53, 61
lingual, xiii, 2, 10, 14, 15, 17, 33, 56, 69, 116, 121, 122, 126
lingual gyrus, 14, 15, 69, 121, 126

local efficiency, x, xiii, xv, 2, 4, 27, 33, 34, 88, 105, 118, 121, 122, 124
local neuronal injury, 33
long-distance connectivity, 147
longitudinal analyses, xii
longitudinal analysis, xv, 33, 67, 68, 73, 106
longitudinal changes, xii, xv, 70, 105
longitudinal comparison, xii, 88, 90, 94, 109, 117, 118
longitudinal differences, 70, 82, 83, 85, 91, 111
longitudinal visits, xv, 105, 108
long-term disability, viii, 106
low frequency (LF), 9, 27, 28, 31, 110, 116, 120, 123
low frequency sub-bands, 9, 110
low-frequency activity, 32
low-frequency band, 9, 118

M

machine learning algorithm, 4, 146
magnetic resonance imaging (MRI), v, ix, x, xi, xiv, xv, xvi, 3, 4, 5, 6, 7, 34, 35, 45, 46, 47, 48, 52, 53, 54, 55, 56, 58, 63, 64, 65, 67, 68, 71, 72, 73, 89, 91, 93, 94, 97, 100, 101, 107, 108, 109, 111, 121, 122, 125, 127, 128, 131, 133, 134, 135, 136, 137, 138, 139, 145, 147, 148, 150, 151, 153
matrix size, 6, 73, 109
mean diffusivity (MD), 61, 93, 96, 110, 111, 116, 117, 118, 119, 120, 124, 125, 127
mean FD, 13
mean top decile, 12, 13
mean top quartile, 12, 13, 32
medial orbito-frontal cortex, 56
medial prefrontal cortex (MFPC), 14, 26, 28, 79, 81, 93, 107, 126
medial temporal lobe, viii, 2, 47, 79, 80, 90, 107

medial-orbito frontal cortex, xiii, 1, 13, 15, 30, 33, 121
memory, vii, xii, xvi, 30, 32, 68, 105, 114, 116, 119, 125, 126, 127, 138, 150, 153
mesial temporal cortex, ix, xiv, 45, 49, 51, 52, 121
mesolimbic circuit, 53
metabolism, xiv, 56, 60, 63, 67, 68, 69, 71, 72, 75, 100, 132, 153
microstructural connectivity, xiv, 45, 52, 148
midbrain, 2
middle cingulate, 14, 15, 75, 76, 112, 113, 121, 122
middle cingulum, 113, 124
middle temporal cortex, xiii, 1, 13, 15, 30, 33, 55, 121, 141
middle temporal gyrus, 26, 27, 126
minimal communication distance, 140
mirror mechanism, 138, 146, 149
misperception, 4, 31
MNI space, 110
molecular, v, viii, xi, xiv, xv, 41, 45, 46, 47, 48, 52, 57, 59, 67, 71, 72, 89, 90, 94, 107, 121, 122, 127
molecular imaging, v, ix, xi, xiv, xv, 41, 45, 46, 48, 52, 59, 67, 71, 72, 89, 90, 127
Montreal Neurological Institute (MNI), 8, 110
morbidity and mortality, viii, 106
morphological analysis, 6, 73
morphological atrophy, ix
morphometry analysis, 2
motion artifacts, 32, 77, 78
motion correction, 7, 73
motion restriction, 67, 72, 73, 81, 83
motor, vii, xi, xii, xiii, 1, 2, 3, 4, 5, 6, 7, 9, 10, 13, 15, 16, 17, 18, 19, 20, 21, 22, 26, 30, 31, 32, 33, 38, 46, 53, 54, 55, 74, 75, 76, 78, 80, 82, 83, 84, 85, 86, 90, 91, 107, 112, 113, 114, 115, 116, 119, 121, 122, 124, 125, 128

motor and supplementary motor network, 17, 18, 31, 34
motor area, 18, 74, 75, 76, 114, 122, 124
motor control, 3, 125
motor cortex, 2, 14, 16, 18, 19, 54, 79, 80, 83, 91, 121
motor function, 7, 116, 119
motor impairment, 31
motor network, 3, 31
motor symptoms, 53
motor-sensory circuit, 32
motor-sensory network, 10
movement, xii, xvi, 2, 30, 32, 58, 65, 105, 107, 114, 125, 127
movement disorder, 2, 32, 58, 65, 125
movement speed, 30
MPRAGE, 6, 7, 72, 73, 75, 109, 139
MRI/PET, ix, x, xi, xv, 5, 48, 67, 71, 94, 108, 121, 128, 153
multi-circuit dysregulation, xi, xiv, 67, 71
multimodal imaging, x
multimodal integration, 46
multimodal MRI/PET, 72, 109
multiomics, 57
multiparametric imaging, xv, 39, 65, 68, 93, 105, 127
multiparametric quantification, xi, xiv, 46, 56
multiparametric quantifications, 56
multiple comparison corrections, 8
multiple sclerosis, 38, 39, 107, 130
multi-slice, 18, 80, 82
multi-variate pattern analysis (MVPA), 92
mutual inhibition, 32
myelin, viii, 7, 31, 41, 107, 128
myelin content, 31, 41
myelin map, 7

N

negative association, 32, 56

network connectivity, 18, 48, 69, 96, 97, 99, 121
network integration, 11, 33, 86, 91, 110, 118
network integration and specialization, 11, 91, 110
network rerouting, xi, xiii, 2, 34, 124
neural activity, 23, 25, 26, 27, 30, 62, 110, 118, 127
neural circuits, xv, 105, 108
neural oscillations, 31
neurocognitive disorder, 68
neurodegenerative disease, 1, iii, viii, x, xi, 39, 46, 56, 64, 65, 96, 128, 153
neurodegenerative disorder, vii, 46, 68
neuroimaging applications, viii
neuroinflammation, 57, 64
neurologic applications, 57
neurological diseases, xi, xiv, 45, 54, 56
neuronal activation, 9
neuronal activity, ix, xv, 3, 9, 31, 33, 105, 124, 128
neuropathological burden, ix, xiv, xv, 67, 71, 94
neuropathological mechanism, xiv, 46, 106
neuropathological quantification, 69
neurophysiology, 57
neuroprotection, 124
neuroprotective, 47
neuropsychiatric disorders, 47
neuropsychiatric problems, vii, 46
neuropsychological profile dysexecution, 68
neuropsychological tests, 93
neurovascular dysfunction, 106, 129
nigrosome-1, xiv, 2, 3, 35, 45, 47, 52
nigrosome-1 imaging, 47
nigrosome-1 territory, xiv, 45, 52
nigrostriatal degeneration, 3
nigrostriatal pathway, 48
non-parametric permutation, 7
normal controls (NC), ix, x, xi, xii, xiii, xiv, 1, 5, 6, 12, 13, 14, 15, 16, 17, 18, 19, 20, 21, 22, 23, 24, 25, 26, 27, 29, 30, 31, 32,

33, 45, 49, 50, 51, 52, 72, 74, 75, 76, 77, 78, 82, 83, 84, 88, 90, 91, 92, 94, 95, 121, 122
normalization, 6, 7, 73, 77, 78, 110, 142, 147
normalization error, 77, 78, 147
number of volumes, 6, 73, 109

O

occipital projection, 23, 32
occipitofrontal fasciculus, viii, 138
OFF state, 54
ON state, 54
opercularis, 114, 115, 122, 124, 145
optimal accuracy, 29
optimal performance, 12
orbitofrontal cortex, ix, xiv, 15, 31, 45, 49, 51, 52, 53, 74, 75, 122, 126, 131
orbitofrontal-amygdala connectivity, 92
outlier screening, 7, 74
over-activity, 124

P

paracingulate gyrus, 70
parahippocampus, 56
paramagnetic iron, 3
parietal lobe, xiv, 45, 52, 113
Parkinson's Progression Markers Initiative (PPMI), xi, 5, 48, 72
Parkinsonism, 32, 40, 41, 46, 47, 59, 60, 61, 102
pars opercularis, 138, 143, 144, 147
pars triangularis, 138, 142, 144
pathophysiological processes, 56
pathophysiology, 3, 57
pathophysiology of the disease, 3
PD from general cohort (GPD), xiii, xiv, 1, 4, 5, 6, 8, 12, 13, 14, 16, 18, 21, 22, 23,

25, 27, 28, 29, 30, 31, 32, 33, 45, 49, 50, 51, 52, 53, 121
PD patients, vii, xi, xiii, 2, 3, 4, 12, 13, 14, 15, 18, 19, 20, 24, 26, 27, 28, 30, 31, 32, 41, 47, 49, 50, 53, 54
percentage reduction, 49, 50, 52
perception, 31
perfusion, 47, 58, 69, 100, 102, 106, 108, 146
perfusion network, 47
perfusion volume fraction, 108
PET/MRI, v, viii, xi, xiv, 45, 46, 53, 54, 55, 56, 63, 64, 65, 68, 127, 135, 136, 153
pharmacotherapy, 53
phenotypic association, 137
phenotypic data, xii, xvi, 137, 139, 141
physiological noise, 9
PiB tracer, 56, 72, 74, 75
planning and execution, 32, 70
PM group, 6, 13, 49, 52
polygenetic, viii, 138
polynomial function, 12
pons, 3, 64, 90, 112, 113, 122
postcentral gyrus, 14, 121
posterior cingulate, 8, 32, 47, 81, 83, 85, 91, 114, 124
posterior cingulate cortex (PCC), 8, 47, 48
posterior limb, 77, 89
posterior putamen, 13, 15, 16, 18, 49, 50, 121
postural instability, 46
power spectrum, 9
precentral gyrus, 15, 126
precuneus, viii, 3, 10, 17, 47, 56, 69, 70, 75, 76, 90, 142
prediction, xii, xvi, 96, 128, 137, 146, 148
premotor cortex, 93, 107
presymptomatic FTD, 70
prevalence, vii, 39, 46
prevention, 57, 85, 128
primary motor cortex, 54

primary progressive aphasia (PPA), vii, 68, 94
primary tracts, 125
primary visual cortex, 14, 74, 75, 90
probabilistic tract template, 110
prodromal (PM), xi, xiii, xiv, 1, 2, 4, 5, 6, 12, 13, 16, 18, 21, 22, 23, 24, 25, 29, 30, 31, 32, 33, 42, 45, 46, 49, 51, 52, 53, 62, 73, 102, 121, 130
prodromal patients, xi, 4, 32
prodromal stage, 2, 6, 25
progressive degeneration, 92
progressive disability, 53
putamen, vii, ix, xi, xiii, xiv, 2, 4, 8, 13, 15, 16, 18, 22, 24, 26, 32, 34, 45, 46, 47, 49, 50, 52, 53, 74, 75, 121, 122, 126
putamen-mesolimbic, vii, 4, 22, 33

Q

quadratic fitting (QP), 12, 29
quantifications, x, xi, xiv, 45, 46, 48, 56, 88, 121, 122, 128
quantitative metrics, xi, xiii, 2, 34
quantitative susceptibility mapping (QSM), 3, 35, 58, 59
quantitative VMHC, xiii, 2, 74

R

radial basis function (RBF), 12, 29
radial diffusivity (RD), 110, 111, 116, 117, 118, 119, 120, 122, 124, 127
radial space, 13, 116, 119
random network, 12
rate, vii, 46
realignment, 73
rectus, 15, 49, 51, 52, 56, 121
red nucleus, 14, 15, 16, 18, 90, 121
reference image, 6, 73, 109
reflective mentalization, 138

regional volume, 140, 141, 142
region-of-interest (ROI), xiv, 11, 13, 45, 48, 50, 51, 52, 91, 111
registration, 56, 110
regression analysis, 10
relative global efficiency, 27, 121
relative local efficiency, 12, 87, 88
relaxing conditions, x, xii, 72, 76, 78, 84, 85, 86, 87, 88
resting state functional connectivity (RSFC), 3, 4, 8, 9, 18, 25, 26, 27, 28, 32, 37, 74, 96, 97, 100
resting state network (RSN), vii, 9, 37, 42, 69, 96
resting-state (RS), vii, xi, xiv, 3, 4, 5, 6, 7, 8, 9, 13, 32, 36, 37, 38, 39, 41, 42, 46, 67, 68, 69, 70, 71, 72, 73, 76, 78, 84, 85, 86, 87, 88, 93, 95, 96, 97, 98, 101, 102, 109, 110, 118, 123, 134, 135, 139
resting-state (RS)-fMRI, xi, xiv, 3, 4, 7, 8, 9, 13, 32, 67, 70, 71, 72, 73, 76, 78, 84, 85, 86, 87, 88, 93, 118, 123
resting-state fMRI, 46, 68, 97, 102, 134
resting-state functional connectivity (RSFC), 3, 4, 8, 9, 18, 25, 26, 27, 28, 32, 74, 96
restricted interests, viii, 138
revised autism diagnostic interview (ADI-R), 138, 139, 141, 145
reward seeking, 32
right frontoparietal network, 70
right medial orbital olfactory, 141, 142
rigidity, vii, 11, 46
ronto-parietal network (FPN), vii, xi, 4, 10, 17, 18, 19, 31, 32, 33, 34, 69
root mean square (RMS), 13
RSFC networks, 25, 32
RS-fMRI, xi, xiv, 3, 4, 7, 8, 9, 13, 32, 67, 70, 71, 72, 73, 76, 78, 84, 85, 86, 87, 88, 93, 118, 123

S

S4, x, xv, 9, 27, 31, 88, 105, 110, 118, 121, 122, 123, 124
S5, 9, 88, 110, 123
sagittal striatum, 76, 77, 89, 122
salience network, vii, 4, 10, 17, 69, 70, 76, 78, 91, 92, 96, 115, 122, 124
sclerosis, viii, 107
seed-based analysis, 7
seed-based approach, 69
seeds, 8, 10, 25, 26, 145
selected imaging features, 141
sensitivity, ix, 10, 12, 93, 95, 146
sensorimotor network, vii, 3
sensory, 10, 17, 26, 112, 113, 115, 116, 119, 122, 124, 125
signal to noise ratio (SNR), 11
simultaneous PET/MRI, 56, 63, 127, 135
sleep behavior disorder, 3
slow onset, 68
slow wave S4 band, 9
slow wave S5 band, 9
slowness, vii, ix, 32, 46, 124
slowness of movement, vii, 46
slowness of speed, ix
slow-wave, x, xv, 9, 28, 31, 88, 105, 106, 110, 118, 123, 124
slow-wave sub-band S4, x, xv, 118, 124
small vessel disease (SVD), viii, xv, 105, 106, 108, 126, 129, 130, 131, 132, 133
small-worldness, x, xiii, xv, 1, 2, 5, 9, 11, 27, 29, 68, 71, 86, 87, 88, 89, 91, 105, 106, 110, 118, 123, 124, 126, 138, 140, 146, 147
small-worldness analysis, x, xiii, xv, 2, 27, 29, 91, 105, 106, 110, 124, 146
small-worldness factor, xiii, 2, 12, 27, 29, 87, 88, 89, 91, 118, 123
small-worldness network analysis, 9, 126, 138, 146, 147

social and learning abilities, 139
social behavior, 68
social context network, 92
social interactions, 138
social responsiveness scale (SRS), 139, 141, 145
social skills, viii, 138
somatosensory cortex, 113, 114
somatosensory integration, 116
sparsity levels, 11
spatial normalization, 7, 147
spatial resolution, 6, 47, 73, 109, 139
specific network pattern, 7
specificity, 12, 93, 146
speech deficits, viii, 138
spin-echo EPI, 73, 110
spontaneous brain activity, 9, 135
staging, 46, 94
statistical analysis, 7
statistical comparisons, 15, 18, 49, 88
statistical parametric mapping (SPM), 73
stereotypical repetitive movements, viii, 138
stereotypy association, 70
striatal binding ratio, ix, xiv, 45, 46, 48, 49, 50, 121
striatal binding ratio (SBR), ix, xi, xiv, 45, 46, 48, 49, 50, 52, 53, 121
striatal dopamine transporters (DAT), ix, xi, xiv, 45, 47, 48, 49, 50, 52, 53, 121
striatum, xiv, 2, 3, 14, 15, 30, 33, 45, 47, 49, 50, 52, 74, 75, 76, 77, 89, 107, 121, 122, 126, 148
stroke, viii, 106, 107, 108, 114, 125, 127, 128, 132, 133, 136
stroop task, 126
structural changes, 107
structural conductivity, 8
structural connectivity, xi, 94, 138
structural MRI, 72, 109, 130, 138
structural network, 108, 134
sub-band S4, 28
subcortical circuits, viii, 138

sub-networks, 10, 151
substantia nigra (SN), vii, ix, xi, xii, xiii, xiv, 1, 2, 3, 4, 6, 13, 14, 15, 16, 18, 30, 33, 35, 40, 45, 46, 47, 52, 53, 58, 59, 69, 92, 114, 115, 121, 122, 124, 133
subthalamic nucleus (STN), 3, 54, 61, 62
superior frontal, x, xvi, 14, 15, 16, 18, 75, 76, 78, 79, 81, 90, 107, 112, 113, 114, 121, 122, 137, 143, 144
superior frontal gyrus (SFG), 107, 112, 113, 122
superior frontal region, x, 90, 143, 144
superior longitudinal fasciculus (SLF), 110, 112, 116, 118, 120, 124, 125
superior parietal lobe, 14, 90
superior parietal lobule, 3
superior temporal gyrus, viii, 69, 138
supplementary motor, xi, xiii, 2, 3, 10, 13, 15, 16, 17, 18, 19, 20, 21, 30, 31, 33, 55, 76, 78, 79, 82, 83, 91, 107, 116, 121, 122, 124, 126
supplementary motor area (SMA), xi, 2, 3, 14, 18, 107, 116, 122, 124, 126
support vector machine (SVM), 12, 29, 30
supracalcarine, 69
supramarginal, 54, 55, 56, 92, 142
supramarginal gyrus, 54, 55, 56
supratentorial volume, 140, 142, 143
supratentorial volume normalization, 140, 142
susceptibility weighted imaging (SWI), 47, 58
swallow tail sign, ix, xiii, xiv, 1, 2, 13, 14, 15, 30, 33, 45, 46, 52, 121
swallow tail sign signature, ix, xiii, 1, 13, 30, 33, 52
swallow tail signs, 14, 15, 121
system breakdown, 128
systematic analysis, 86, 88, 108, 118, 123
systematic coordination, 32
systematic integration, x, xv, 94, 105, 124
systematic investigation, 9

T

task-based fMRI, 146
task-positive networks, 8
tau, 48, 57, 64, 69
tau burden, 57
template matching, xi, 10
template networks, 10
template space, 111
template-based ICA, 9
temporal, v, vii, ix, x, xi, xii, xiii, xiv, xv, xvi, 2, 3, 9, 10, 14, 15, 16, 17, 18, 19, 24, 25, 30, 31, 32, 34, 37, 45, 49, 51, 52, 53, 56, 67, 68, 70, 74, 75, 76, 77, 78, 79, 80, 81, 83, 84, 85, 89, 90, 92, 94, 106, 107, 110, 112, 113, 116, 118, 120, 121, 122, 124, 125, 126, 128, 137, 142, 144, 146
temporal atrophy, 69, 126
temporal cortex, xi, xiii, 2, 14, 15, 16, 17, 18, 31, 34, 49, 51, 52, 56, 76, 78, 90, 92, 121, 122
temporal lobe, 3, 56, 106, 107
temporal network, 10, 17
temporal part, 110, 116, 118, 120, 125
temporal projection, 32
thalamic network, xi, xiii, 2, 17, 18, 31, 82, 85
thalamocortical, vii, 4, 19, 32, 102
thalamo-cortical connectivity, 10
thalamo-cortical networks, 10, 17, 33, 34
thalamus, xiii, 2, 3, 8, 14, 15, 18, 19, 26, 27, 28, 30, 32, 34, 47, 53, 75, 76, 78, 89, 90, 91, 92, 112, 113, 114, 115, 121, 122, 124, 126
theory of mind (ToM), 92, 99, 150
thorough analysis, x
tissue microenvironment, 107
topological organization, 126
TR/TE, 6, 73, 109

Index

tract-based, xii, xv, 73, 105, 106, 108, 110, 111, 116, 117, 128
tract-based quantification, xii
tract-based spatial statistics (TBSS), 73, 76, 77, 106, 110, 112, 117, 125
tract-specific, 110
transcranial magnetic stimulation (TMS), 54
transitional stage, 31
treatment, 33, 42, 47, 53, 54, 58, 61, 62, 93, 94, 153
treatment efficacy, 33, 47
tremor, vii, 2, 5, 30, 32, 40, 46
triangularis, 114, 122, 144, 145, 147
typical functional networks, 8
typically developing (TD), vii, viii, x, xii, xvi, 57, 68, 101, 137, 138, 139, 141, 142, 146, 147

U

unbalanced networks, 146
uncinate fasciculus, xii, xvi, 93, 105, 106, 107, 110, 112, 116, 118, 119, 120, 122, 124, 127
unified Parkinson's disease rating scale (UPDRS), 5, 6, 32, 53, 54
unilateral, 63, 77, 78

V

VABS interpersonal skills, 145
VABS social skill scores, 144
VaD, viii, ix, xii, xv, 105, 106, 107, 108, 109, 121, 122, 125, 126, 127, 128
vascular cognitive disorder (VCD), 106, 129
vascular dementia (VaD), v, viii, ix, xii, xv, 105, 106, 107, 108, 109, 111, 114, 121, 122, 125, 126, 127, 128, 129, 131, 133, 135
vascular dementia of Binswanger type (SVaD-BT), 125, 126, 133

ventral striatum (VST), 14, 15, 47, 121
ventral tegmental area (VTA), 47
verbal, 140, 150
vesicular monoamine transporter, ix, xiv, 45, 46, 47
vesicular monoamine transporter type 2 (VMAT2), ix, xi, xiv, 45, 47, 48, 49, 51, 52, 60, 121
Vinland adaptive behavior scale (VABS), 139, 141, 144, 145
virtual reality paradigm, 53
visual cortex, 18, 20, 47, 74, 75, 76, 114, 122, 124
visual networks, 9, 10, 17, 33
VMAT2 densities, xiv, 45, 48, 49, 52, 121
VMHC computation, 77, 113
volume, 63, 141, 142, 143, 146, 147
volumetry, xii, xvi, 137, 140, 141, 146, 147
voxel based morphometry (VBM), ix, x, xi, 7, 13, 15, 30, 40, 55, 72, 73, 74, 75, 102, 109, 112, 113, 121, 122, 133
voxel-mirrored homotopic correlation (VMHC), ix, xi, xiii, xiv, xv, 1, 2, 7, 12, 14, 15, 16, 18, 23, 24, 25, 26, 29, 30, 32, 33, 67, 68, 71, 76, 77, 78, 86, 89, 105, 106, 110, 113, 114, 121, 122, 124, 126, 127, 128
voxel-wise, 8, 33, 39, 73

W

Wallerian degeneration, xii, xvi, 106, 116, 120, 125, 127
white matter (WM), viii, ix, xii, xv, xvi, 7, 51, 76, 77, 78, 89, 93, 96, 97, 98, 99, 100, 101, 103, 105, 106, 107, 108, 110, 111, 112, 116, 119, 125, 127, 128, 130, 131, 132, 133, 137, 140, 141, 142, 143, 146, 147
white matter bundle, 112
white matter injury, 106, 128

white matter integrity, ix, xii, xvi, 89, 93, 106, 111, 116, 119, 127
white matter skeleton template, 110
white matter volume, x, xii, xvi, 137, 143
whole brain, 7, 8, 73, 117
whole-brain parcellation, 11
WM abnormalities, 108
WM hyperintensities (WMH), 107, 125
WM injury, viii, ix, 126
WM integrity, 107, 125
working memory, viii, 69

Z

Zarit Burden Interview (ZBI), 106
Z-value, 12, 23, 24, 25, 26, 27, 28, 29